TEENs

Teens
Easing
Exam
Nerves

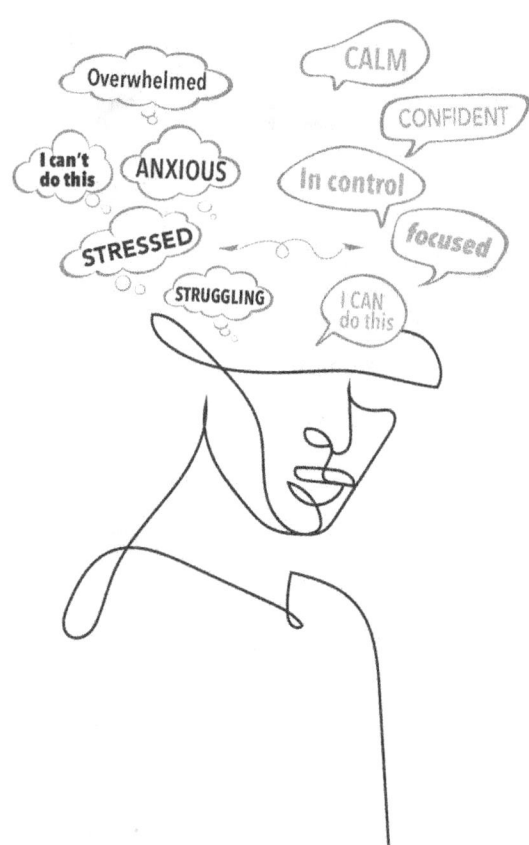

TEENs

Teens
Easing
Exam
Nerves

Alison Middleton Timms

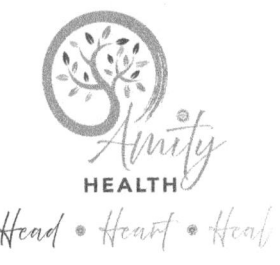

TEENS: TEENS EASING EXAM NERVES
© 2024 Alison Middleton Timms
All rights reserved.

Paperback ISBN: 978-1-7385077-0-2
Ebook ISBN: 978-1-7385077-1-9

Images by Hound Dog Creatives

Author's Note

If you are worried about a fellow student's or your child's wellbeing and safety, then please do talk to them about your concerns directly. (See the section about self-harm and suicide for tips on how to do this.) This may involve alerting another adult in a better position to help when someone we know is really struggling. You are not telling tales or stepping out of line here. We all have a duty to look out for each other.

'I'm not afraid of storms for I am learning to sail my ship.'

—Louisa May Alcott

Dedication

This book is dedicated to all students out there. I wish you all the best and really hope this book helps you nail those exams. (I wish I'd had access to such tools and resources in my time.) To Alex my son, one of those students (sorry I am an embarrassing mum!), best of luck and know I am so proud of you, whatever your results.

Acknowledgements

In honour and thanks to my late parents too for all their loving support. Being a parent during exam time is not much fun, which I especially realise now being a mum of a teenager myself!

Thank you also to all my family and friends who have encouraged and supported me along the way. I am grateful to you all.

With special thanks to:
Eden Gruger, author and mentor, for guiding me through the whole process of writing a book and keeping me on track! Writing a book

Acknowledgements

is one thing but getting it published is quite another challenge, as I have found out.

Laurenne Dorgan of Hound Dog Creatives for all her wonderful creativity on my website, social media, and designing my cover supporting the launch of TEENs and being on the journey with me, keeping me going with our daily catch ups. I have a friend for life!

Chrystal Hill, thank you for all your wonderful support and guidance. I wouldn't be where I am today without your support and friendship, so eternally grateful to you.

Liz Clark of Lizzie@Bizziepa for all her ideas and enthusiasm at helping market the book.

Sarah Holroyd of Sleeping Cat Books for all her patience editing and formating TEENs.

Contents

Who Is This Book For? 13
Students..13
Parents 15
Teachers/Head of Years/Directors of Student Wellbeing/Pastoral Care/Exam Officers/Educators 16
Ways to Use This Book 18
About Me 20
Preface: You Are Not Alone 24

Part One: Background 27
Exam Anxiety: What It Is 29
Good stress versus bad stress 30
Stress Overload: Overflowing Cup & Snowball Analogies. 32
What makes us stressed? 32
3 Key States: Safe and Social, Fight or Flight, & Freeze Modes 33
Where are you at? 37
Why do some of us seem to cope better than others? 39
Personality and Ability to Cope with Stressful Situations. 41

Type A and Type B Personality Theory.......41
Helper, Achiever, Perfectionist, Anxiety,
Controller Behaviour Patterns......................43
The Highly Sensitive Person (HSP) 46
Neurodivergence... 50
ACES 51
COVID 2020 52
Trauma with a little 't'.................................53
Summary of Part One......................... 57

Part Two: Solutions 59
Introduction 61
The 5 Ps..62
Exam Preparation and Revision 63
**Mindset and Change the Way You
Think & Feel Tools 75**
Emotions and Feelings 103
**Tools to Get Us Back into Safe and
Social 115**
Mindfulness, Meditation & Breathwork..... 115
EFT/Emotional Freedom Technique (also
known as Tapping)..130
Journalling & Automatic or Free Writing . 142
Anxiety-Busting Diet 149
Exercise 158
Grounding 163
Sleep...164
Essential Oils/Aromatherapy 167

Crystals for Anxiety & Stress Relief 168
Calming Basket... 171
Seeking Professional Help.................. 172
Clinical hypnotherapy 172
Cognitive Behavioural therapy (CBT) 173
Self-harm & Suicidal Thoughts 174
Useful UK Contact Numbers 180
Summary of Part Two......................... 184
Easing Exam Nerves Daily Protocol 186

Conclusion and Moving Forwards ... 187
Resources 189
Anti-Exam-Anxiety Smoothie..................... 190
Comforting Bedtime Golden Tea/Latte 192
Extra Reading Materials, References and Resources 194
About the Author 223

Who Is This Book For?

Whilst this book is primarily written directly to and for students and I use the term 'you' throughout for ease of reading, my hope is that this is also a practical guide and reference for parents and teachers too. So please exchange 'you' for 'they' as appropriate.

Students
Are you a student with exams looming and feeling the emotional and physical strain like a heavy cloud hanging over you? Maybe you are doing okay but a friend is struggling. Do feel free to point them in the way of this book.

Are you feeling:
- Overwhelmed, stressed, anxious or panicky?
- Sick with nerves, stomach churning?
- Heart beating faster, having panic attacks even?
- Unable to fall, or stay, sleep?
- Constantly worried?

Afraid that:
- You won't remember anything at all?
- Your mind will go blank and you'll feel paralysed?
- You won't perform at your best?
- You won't get the grades you need to get into the college or university of your choice?
- You might not do as well as your friends and peers?
- You won't live up to your parents' and teachers' expectations?
- You won't live up to your own?

Want to:
- Feel in control?
- Feel confident and calm?
- Take the exams in your stride?
- Be able to calm yourself down quickly and easily?

- Be motivated to study and concentrate?
- Remember all you have learned?
- Do the best you can do and know you are capable of?
- Come out with the results you deserve?

Parents

Are you a parent of a student who is struggling with severe exam nerves and anxiety?

Are you yourself feeling:
- Stressed, overwhelmed, constantly worried and anxious about how best to support your child?
- Lost as to what to do next or to whom to turn?
- That you are treading on eggshells?
- Not sure what to do or say?
- Worried about how to manage the situation, and not wanting to make it worse?
- Concerned your child won't perform to the best of their abilities, get the grades they need and what that might mean for their future?
- Worried that their friends may judge them and your child may feel isolated or even be bullied?

Then you are in the right place!

Want to see your child:
- Take exams in their stride?
- Be able to focus on revision and during the exams themselves?
- Have access to tools that help them feel less anxious (and you can support them with)?
- Get the results they desire and deserve?

Teachers/Head of Years/Directors of Student Wellbeing/Pastoral Care/Exam Officers/Educators

Are you seeing:
- Students struggling with exam anxiety?
- Students not performing to their capacity?
- Students getting lower grades than they are capable of and deserve?

Want to:
- See your students achieve the results they are looking for?
- Have access to tools and resources that can help you support them to take revision and exams in their stride?

Who Is This Book For?

- Know you are doing everything you can to help them through a challenging time?

Whatever age you are, and whether you are facing exams, either in a supporting role or going through them yourself, there will be something here for you. These tips will also be helpful for those who are suffering from nerves, auditioning for music, dance and drama places, for those taking their driving test or for those undergoing university or job interviews too.

Ways to Use This Book

You might want to read this book from cover to cover, or dip in and out of various chapters as you feel called to. Everything here is an invitation. All I ask is that you read this book with curiosity and take from it what resonates and works for you.

What you will learn from this book:
- An understanding of anxiety and stress.
- Why some students may be more prone to anxiety than others.
- Ways to make revision even more effective.
- How to shift into the right mindset to take revision and exams in your stride.

Ways to Use This Book

- Practical, quick, and easy strategies and tools that can instantly calm the nervous system.

The resources you will learn here will serve you for life, not just at exam times. Whenever you feel anxiety and worry creeping in, you'll be able to feel back in control again, regaining your balance and perspective.

About Me

I was a senior Human Resources (HR) manager in the legal sector for twenty years before becoming Global Group Head of Talent & Development for a premium international school's organisation, which now has over sixty schools worldwide.

In 2014 I had a major health scare, which was a massive wakeup call and made me reassess my life. I believe the illness was due in part to stress. The pressure that had built up over many years just got to me. It was partly the pressure I put on myself as the main breadwinner in the family, partly

About Me

pressure to be the best employee and the best wife, mum and daughter. So I was forced to really look at my life. I reclaimed my health, training in a variety of mind-body therapies that enabled me to become well again. Through this, it became clear to me that, in order to perform at our best, we need to be physically, mentally and emotionally balanced.

I was blown away by what I learned and, especially, with how amazing it can be to work with the power of our subconscious mind. It enabled me to question the thoughts I had about myself and the world. Over time I have been able to reprogramme my limiting patterns and beliefs. I changed my view of life and what I wanted to do going forwards.

Fast forward a few years and I am now an experienced Mind and Body Wellbeing Practitioner, specialising in anxiety, stress, trauma and resilience. I support teens and adults to become their best versions of themselves and to thrive, no matter what is going on in their lives.

Partnering with my clients, we look at the root cause of what they are struggling with – be it confidence issues, trauma recovery, addictive patterns, anxiety, depression or relationship issues. Together, we look at what is holding them back, their beliefs about the world and life, their patterns of behaviour and reactions to events. We then work towards fulfilling their goals in life so that they feel comfortable in their skin and become the best versions of themselves.

I absolutely love what I do, as I get so much joy seeing people transform and grow. And I can think of no greater honour than to help equip our younger generation with tools that will stand them in good stead, whatever they face in life.

This book is fuelled by my genuine desire and passion to make going through exams a less challenging time for all concerned. Still today I am haunted by the nightmare of getting into an exam room, opening the paper and fearing I cannot answer any of the questions. As I write this, I'm experiencing that same dread and sickness at the pit of the stomach, and I haven't taken an exam for years!

About Me

My son sat his GCSEs (General Certificate of Secondary Education) in 2022. He is usually a calm, balanced, happy-go-lucky teenager, yet even he felt the pressure. At the time he was staying away from home and rang me one evening in the week leading up to the exams, quite concerned because he was having heart palpitations and the beginning of a panic attack. One of the worst things about being a parent is seeing or hearing when our children suffer and us not knowing how to best help or support them.

Preface: You Are Not Alone

I want you to know that you are not alone. Exam anxiety is very real, and you are not the only one experiencing it, though it might feel that way.

Approximately three million pupils in the UK sit exams each summer, and according to ChildLine's Exam Stress Survey, 96% of the 1,300 who completed the survey felt anxious about exams and revision (Mental Healthy website, *Pressure of exams causing worrying levels of anxiety in students*).

PREFACE: YOU ARE NOT ALONE

In March 2020, the Childrens' Commissioner asked almost 2,000 eight- to seventeen-year-olds about stress. Two thirds (66%) of students felt most stressed about homework or exams, ahead of worrying about what other people think of them (39%) and bullying (25%) (Children's Commissioner website, *Children and stress, what's worrying them most*).

On further questioning, it was found that this anxiety came from:
- Fear of failure and letting oneself down.
- Pressure from teachers to do well.
- Fear of being at the bottom of the class and feeling stupid or embarrassed because of it.
- Fear of having to move down a grade or repeat a year.
- Fear of not getting into college or university.
- Fear of being bullied by peers.

In my experience as an exam invigilator in the UK (called a 'proctor' in the US), schools are receiving more access requests from individual students for extra time, to be in smaller exam rooms and to be able to go out and have rest breaks when they feel overwhelmed. I have calmed students who have had panic attacks before or during their exams. One student even sat with a bucket next to her, as she was physically sick during every exam.

Many universities, I am delighted to see, are now moving away from exams as their main assessment tool to using broader course work assessments and presentations.

You will be pleased to hear that exams are not a massive feature in the world of work. In my twenty-five years in the corporate world, apart from my own Professional CIPD (HR) qualifications and the occasional psychometric tests for promotions and new job roles, I haven't had to undertake any. So that is good news.

Exams, however, are a part of school life for now, and here you will find proven strategies that will enable you not only to cope but to thrive.

Part One:
Background

Exam Anxiety: What It Is

So, let's dive in. The university of Maryland Medical Center defines anxiety as "a persistent feeling of fear, unease and worry."

Anxiety is not the same as fear, though sometimes the two terms are used interchangeably.

Fear is our natural response to a potential threat – think of walking in a forest and coming across a big grizzly bear. We would call this an acute episode where the fear usually dissipates and disappears after the threat is over and the grizzly bear has gone away. It is usually short-lived.

Anxiety is a persistent worry about something that may or may not happen in the future. So looming exams fall under this. Your body reacts physically and emotionally in the same way as if that threat is here and now. There are a lot of 'what if' worries. *What if I can't remember anything? What if I don't get the results I need?* When that worry is constant and persistent, we go into a chronic state of stress or alert. Chronic is when something persistently affects our day-to-day life. It doesn't go away.

Good stress versus bad stress

Yes, you heard me correctly; not all stress is bad for us. A certain level of stress and anxiety is perfectly normal and, actually, helpful. It is needed for us to be focused, motivated, organised and to make good decisions. Those butterflies before an exam, presentation or a race are normal signs that our body is getting us prepared and ready to perform at the top of our game.

When there is not enough stress, we can become apathetic, bored and unmotivated.

Exam Anxiety: What It Is

When there is too much stress over too long a period, however, we can feel scattered, disorganised, burnt out and exhausted. Our bodies and minds are no longer able to function optimally. We may experience physical symptoms such as headaches, and be more prone to coughs, colds, bugs and viruses due to our immune system being weaker. We may lose our appetite, not be able to sleep and feel tired.

Stress Overload: Overflowing Cup & Snowball Analogies

Think of a cup that reaches its limit and suddenly overflows. Or you might prefer to think of stress like a snowball rolling down a mountain, gradually building in size and speed until it has a momentum all its own and is virtually impossible to control.

What makes us stressed?

There are many times in life that external events, outside of our control – like moving school or house, losing a job or relationship, being ill or a new baby in the family – cause us stress.

Other factors, such as taking on too much work or too many activities or leaving it to the last minute to complete a homework assignment or revise for a test, are also stressful, but these are more within our control. You can do something about these. By becoming aware that this is your tendency you can take action. You might decide not to do that extra class after school and to perhaps tackle that piece of homework instead, which is not due in until the end of the week. This gives you a bit more breathing space and can take the pressure off.

Much of this book is about understanding your own tendencies and repeating patterns. By having that awareness, you can take back control and ease the pressure and anxiety.

3 Key States: Safe and Social, Fight or Flight, & Freeze Modes

It has been shown that our bodies, and more importantly our nervous systems, are always in one of three key states:

- **Safe and Social (relaxed mode):** This state is also known as *rest and digest*. Your nervous system is calm. You interact and connect with family and friends, going out socialising and enjoying yourself and their company. You are also happy being on your own, able to switch off and relax. Your breathing, heart rate and digestion are all normal. You are able to be fully present in the moment, not worrying about the past or fretting about the future. You feel grounded and safe. In this state your body and mind can rest, heal and repair. Even if you experience an episode of acute stress (remember the grizzly bear), this is the state to which you want to return immediately after the threat is over.

- **Fight or Flight state (mobilised mode):** In this state, our bodies have detected a threat and are on alert, automatically primed for action. Your system is gearing up to fight or run from that grizzly bear. You may feel 'wired', which is the increased levels of adrenaline and cortisol in your system. It can be difficult to relax, even when your body is inactive. Your heart rate goes up, and your breathing becomes shallow. You may feel the need to run to the loo – your bowels might turn to water, or you might vomit. This is to get rid of the contents of your stomach as you can't afford to waste energy on digesting food. All your energy is going to fighting or running for your life.

In this hypervigilant state, we are prone to see situations and people as dangerous, even when they may be neutral. An example of this might be snapping at someone who asks a question or pushing someone away who is genuinely trying to help you. This is your body in the height of survival mode. And, of course, if we were to meet that grizzly bear, then we would want our body to kick into this gear. We just do not want to be stuck in this mode for too long. With exam anxiety it can feel as though the threat is constant. It never ends. And it can seem impossible to get back to feeling *safe and social*. I am going to show you how you can. And it is easier than you might think.

- **Freeze state (immobilised mode):** In this state, in the grizzly bear scenario, our body automatically decides to freeze or 'play dead'. In the wild, animals will often do this so the predator will decide that they are not worth bothering with and turn their attention elsewhere. In this state our bodies shut down, and may become rigid or limp, with our breathing slowed right down.

Usually once the initial threat is over, we would expect to return to *safe and social* mode. With the lead-up to exams and the exam period itself, the prolonged stress may mean that you might, through panic, go into freeze mode and not find it easy to come out of it.

This might lead to withdrawing from family and friends, feeling a bit numb and apathetic or not really being motivated to do anything. You might find it hard to think or function, or you might have low energy. In some cases, you may *dissociate*. This is when you feel disconnected or have literally escaped from yourself. You don't really feel as if you are in your body. You may feel floaty, spaced out, and it may seem as if everything is happening to someone else and you are not really in this world. You might feel more like an observer of life, not a full participant.

We all experience this to a certain extent from time to time. Think about driving or cycling somewhere and having no memory of getting there. Or leaving the house and having no awareness of shutting the door or locking up. It is as though we are operating on automatic, without being present. Dissociation can last for a few minutes or hours, or can become a longer-term coping mechanism we adopt to escape a stressful or traumatic situation. If you dissociate to escape from the stress of exams and you do not 'return to yourself' after a time, you are not in the best state to think, concentrate or focus.

I hope you can start to recognise when you might be slipping into or getting stuck in fight, flight or freeze mode. Whilst it is normal to flit between all three states at different times, and maybe even in the same day, the aim is to always return back to *safe and social*.

Where are you at?

I'd just like you to reflect on where you – or the individual you are supporting – are mostly based right now. Which state do you spend most of your time in? Ideally you want to be in *safe and social* most of the time. Are you?

How is exam anxiety affecting you? What symptoms and signs are you experiencing or noticing? I list the most common ones below for ease of reference.

Are you in that fight or flight mode?
- Headaches.
- Loss of the ability to concentrate and focus.
- Feeling tired and wired.
- Unable to sleep.
- Feeling irritable.
- Experiencing mood fluctuations, out bursts, over thinking.
- Experiencing OCD issues.
- Having digestive issues.
- Nail biting.
- Wanting to or actually self-harming (please see separate section at the back of the book on this).

Or are you more in the freeze mode?
- Grappling with avoidance and procrastination.
- Withdrawing from family and friends.
- Generally feeling low, unmotivated and depressed.

At school/college how is this affecting you?
- Struggling to keep up.
- Feeling overwhelmed.
- Missing deadlines.
- Not completing homework.
- Getting lower grades.
- Not able to concentrate in class or focus.
- Withdrawing from friends or socialising at lunch or at break times.

For now, notice where you are with curiosity – no judgement or blame here. This is all important knowledge and awareness about you and your patterns.

Why do some of us seem to cope better than others?

Some people seem to breeze through life without a care in the world, don't they? Whilst others are more affected by stressful events and exams. Why is this? There are many factors at play.

1. Stress load: This is our ability, resources and state to cope with the load on us at the time. This will depend on what other stresses we might be under – for example, at the time of an exam, a family illness or loss, moving home etc.

2. Stress Lens: The way we interpret our experiences and the meaning we give them. For example, if two students narrowly fail a test, one might look at that and say, "*I'm a failure, I'm never going to get the grades I want. What is the point? I am giving up.*" The other student may say, "*I only just missed the mark. I'm so nearly there and I'll make sure next time I get the grade I need. It has shown me where I need to focus.*" Feel the difference? What would be *your* response?

3. Our Stress Signature: This is about our personality and how our bodies are physically, emotionally and mentally wired.

Personality and Ability to Cope with Stressful Situations

Have a think as you read through this next section and what resonates with you.

Type A and Type B Personality Theory

The Type A and Type B personality theory describes two contrasting personality types. (Note: Neither is better than the other.)

Type As are more prone to experience stress. They are seen as competitive, highly organised, ambitious and sometimes impatient. They tend to push themselves to meet deadlines and have high expectations of themselves, often believing that others (parents and teachers) have these same high expectations of them too. All this adds to the pressure they put themselves under to achieve, and even to over-achieve.

In contrast, Type B individuals are generally more easy-going, less intense and frantic, more relaxed and likely to work steadily, being less prone to stress and anxiety.

Where on the scale would you put yourself?

I identify as quite an extreme type A personality. I find it hard to relax. I am very driven, having to finish my work before I can go out and socialise or relax. If working on something and in the flow, I won't concentrate on anything else and can get irritated if interrupted. I hate being late but, knowing this, I compensate by always leaving extra time to get somewhere and to meet deadlines. With regards to exams and revision, it helped me manage my anxiety by starting tasks early.

Knowing I had given myself a lot of time to prepare really helped my confidence. I felt I couldn't have done more. It allowed me to relax and feel calmer, more in control. But it was important to factor in time for breaks and for doing some fun things.

I would say my son veers more towards the Type B end of the scale. He will do things in his own time and is more relaxed regarding deadlines. That puts him under a different level of stress though to get things completed in time. He needs more motivation and encouragement to get going with his revision, and reassurance that he will get there when he feels that it might have been easier to start his work earlier.

Knowing which end of the scale you tend towards can help you plan your approach to revision accordingly.

Helper, Achiever, Perfectionist, Anxiety, Controller Behaviour Patterns

I use these patterns to help my clients understand their motivations and drivers and especially to uncover root limiting beliefs about themselves. When you know what these are you can take action to challenge if they are really true and can work to change them.

The Helper Pattern: Or the *people pleaser* pattern, as I call it, is where you tend to put other people's needs constantly before your own. You might say 'yes' even when you really do not want to do something just to please someone else. Over time you can become increasingly depleted by over giving, often at the detriment of your own health and needs, and you can feel resentment. The underlying core belief here is that you are not worthy of having your needs put first. You want to do well in exams to gain the approval of your parents, family and friends and this adds to the pressure you put on yourself.

The Achiever Pattern: This is where you define yourself by your achievements and so there is a tendency to always strive for more: the higher grade, the next goal in a bid to prove to others and yourself that you are good enough. Exhausting. You want to not only just pass the exam but to get the best grades possible.

The Perfectionist Pattern: Often following on from the Achiever pattern, the Perfectionist is usually highly self-critical, focusing on the details and getting things right, often at the risk of losing sight of the bigger picture. This pattern can be driven by a fear of being judged or failing if you do not do things perfectly. You might not feel good enough just for being you. With regards to exams and revision, there may be a tendency to spend too long on one topic, putting yourself under pressure to complete other subjects. And it never being enough. You might constantly beat yourself up to do more, and you can be prone to burn out if you are not careful.

The Anxiety Pattern: Or the *Worrier*, as I call it, is constantly being on edge, in the head/mind, overthinking and worrying what if x, y, z happens? You may jump to the worst-case scenario. Here, you are really trying to *think* yourself into feeling safe in your own body and/or in the world. You are not able to let your guard down, not able to relax and enjoy life. You may see potential threats in everything. *What if I fail? What if I don't get the grade I need to stay on to the sixth form or to get into the university of my choice?*

The Controller Pattern: This is a close relation to the Anxiety pattern. This is all about wanting to feel safe, feeling a need to control surroundings or others to ensure nothing goes wrong. Needing things to be done a certain way, often taking on massive responsibilities because you are afraid to leave it to others. When things get disrupted – perhaps the revision timetable needs to be shifted – this can cause a meltdown.

Do any of these patterns resonate? Each of these patterns can be standalone or combined (I see myself in all of these to a certain extent). They can spur us on and motivate us, but can exhaust us when lived with day in and day out. Then, when an extra stressor like exams comes along, they can go into overdrive.

The Highly Sensitive Person (HSP)

Are you, or is your child or student, highly sensitive? This is another piece of the jigsaw puzzle in knowing yourself. Equipped with that knowledge about how we react, we can put coping strategies in place.

Through the work of Dr Elaine Aaron in her book *The Highly Sensitive Person*, we know that highly sensitive individuals 'are more aware of the subtleties in their surroundings than others and can become more easily overwhelmed when in a highly stimulating or challenging environment'. Think about big crowds at noisy concerts or football matches and busy shopping centres. HSPs may analyse and process everything around them much more, reflecting on it, elaborating on it, making associations that others may not. So, it follows that in stressful situations and during the lead up to exams and the exams themselves, highly sensitive individuals are likely to be impacted more.

Signs you might be more sensitive may include feeling easily overwhelmed by bright lights, strong smells, textures or hearing sirens; getting rattled or overwhelmed when you have a lot to do; and often, at busy times, needing to take time out away from others.

On a personal note, I have to say that reading Dr Aaron's book was a complete game changer for me. I identified with every trait laid out in her questionnaire and yet I'd had no idea that I was that sensitive.

For me, one of the biggest issues about taking the exams was going into and sitting in the big exam hall surrounded by other students, and the noise and just having other people's energy around me. It was not so bad if I was at the end of a row or at the back or front of the hall, but being in the middle of the hall was quite intimidating and stressful for me. And it is only now that I understand the issue I had. At that time, I just put up with it and struggled through.

Nowadays, this is quite easily rectified. I recommend contacting your school's exams office or your form teacher and talk to them about what access arrangements they may be able to put in place. This might include taking the exam in a smaller room, or having the option of a supervised rest break, or taking time out of the exam if things get a bit too much. Students can leave the exam room and then come back in again when they are ready to resume. The clock on the exam stops when they leave and starts again when they come back in. I know that many of those who have this rest break option do not always need to take it. The comfort is knowing that they have the option.

HSPs can pick up other people's panic or distress and sometimes, if we do not know that we do this, we can mistake it as our own. One thing that can help is to pause and take a step back and to ask 'Is this my energy or it is someone else's that I am feeling?' Do not try to analyse this question; just go with the first answer that comes to you. Yes or no. You can then go on to ask 'What percentage is mine? What percentage is theirs?' The first answer comes from our subconscious mind and is usually our truth. Take a deep breath and just intend to let everyone else's energy go and, with practice, that energy will just dissolve, and you should feel lighter.

A point to note, is that if you, as a parent, identify as highly sensitive, then you may find supporting someone through exams extra challenging – taking on their nerves without perhaps realising it and feeling more on edge yourself. Parents need to ensure they look after themselves. Remember that oxygen mask analogy on an airplane? Put yours on first so you can better take care of everyone else.

Neurodivergence

Students who may have autism spectrum disorder (ASD) or other neurological or developmental conditions such as attention-deficit/hyperactivity disorder (ADHD), ADD, dyslexia or dyspraxia can find being a minority in an educational environment challenging enough. Studies have shown that their rate of stress, anxiety and depression is higher than in the general population, and so exam time is extra challenging.

I am seeing an increasing number of young people with neurodivergence in my practice struggling with anxiety and depression in year eight and year nine (in the UK system).

These children need extra support to explore and process their emotions. (See the *Emotions and Feelings* section in Part Two.) I also suggest that, if you are not in contact with your school about extra support and access arrangements, you do so as early as you can to help ease the extra pressure of exams.

ACES

ACEs are Adverse Childhood Experiences. These are traumatic experiences in childhood, such as going through a separation or divorce, witnessing or experiencing abuse (sexual, emotional or physical), having or living with someone who has a major illness or addiction, or suffering the loss of someone close to you.

Those who experience one or more ACEs are more prone to stress than others, are more likely to self-harm, self-soothe and medicate with addictions (smoking, alcohol, drugs, gambling, shopping) and are more likely to suffer from eating disorders. These reactions are just some of the ways we as individuals seek to escape or cope with the pain of what we have experienced. However, what is initially a helpful ally to cope in the short-term can quickly become an enemy it is hard to escape from.

With regard to exams, students with higher ACE exposure are more likely to repeat a grade and be less engaged with school. Their stress load is already high before adding in exam pressure.

COVID 2020

I class the pandemic as an ACE. It had a massive impact on education and learning and, of course, on exams. So many missed out on direct teaching and exam practice.

We will not know the full impact for many years to come. I have seen the results playing out firsthand in my own practice though. Many young people with anxiety found it extremely difficult to get back into the routine of school again. COVID enabled them to feel very safe at home, and when it was time to return to school, their social anxiety escalated.

The health fears around catching COVID increased the anxiety too. Some of my young clients made the decision that online or home school was a better option for their physical and mental health. Many students, I believe, also suffered burnout from the period of online school too, which in many cases was intense – being on a computer from 8:30 am to 4 pm every day – whilst others were left to their own devices with little or no structure, reliant on parents (often working) to supervise and plug any gaps in learning. This, I believe, has led to some finding it difficult to concentrate in the classroom, which they didn't experience before COVID. Some lost contact with friends and have not been able to develop or re-establish social relationships with others very easily. It has been an unsettling time for all.

Trauma with a little 't'

The events and ACEs above are what I tend to call trauma with a capital or big T.

In my line of work, there is also trauma with a little t. Little t trauma is not so obvious, much more subtle and plays out on the subconscious level. The effects, however, can also be devastating. We are often triggered and react in certain ways but have no idea why.

For me trauma is anything that overwhelms our nervous system, including incidents such as going on stage when we were in primary school for a school concert or performance and forgetting our lines, not being picked for a sports team, or even crying when we were a little baby and for some reason our parent/carer didn't respond immediately.

It does not take much for us when we are young to form 'beliefs' such as 'my needs weren't met', 'I'm not lovable' or 'I am not safe', even if that was never or even near the truth of the matter. Our parent/carer might have been distracted or tending to another child, not neglecting us, but that little younger version of us now holds that as a core belief and we only need a couple more similar incidents to become 'our story', our 'truth' (not necessarily *the* truth). Our subconscious is then on the alert to look out for other experiences to reinforce this belief.

Most of our beliefs or our perceptions, whether true or not, are formed between birth and the age of eight, so we do not always have access to these memories, but they can really affect the way we relate to ourselves and interact with others.

When stressful situations such as exams occur, our fears and beliefs about ourselves that might have been lying deep can come up and make us feel even more insecure. Those beliefs about not being good enough or worthy of doing well may rise to the surface.

I had a young lady who came to me because she found it very hard to speak up in meetings in her job. She was after a promotion at work and this was holding her back. She would get tongue tied, flustered, and go red with embarrassment and fear. We worked together in a one-hour session – that was all it took. When I went back to the root cause of why she couldn't speak up in meetings, a memory (that she consciously hadn't remembered) surfaced. At primary school, she'd been part of a Christmas play and when it came time to speak her lines she froze and couldn't get the words out. The audience laughed and afterwards, off stage, her dad berated her for embarrassing him.

At the time of the play, she was so traumatized that a part of her became stuck or frozen, forming what we call a 'hurt' or 'wounded inner child'. No wonder she did not speak up in meetings. She was subconsciously afraid of being laughed at, criticised and judged. Her subconscious brain was keeping her safe by not exposing her to that situation again. With my guidance, she was quickly and easily able to go in and unfreeze/heal that little girl. And after that one session, she reported back that she no longer had any difficulties speaking up. And she did get that promotion.

So, the good news is that we can move forwards and break habits and patterns of behaviour and reaction.

With regard to exam stress, you may be feeling, like my client above, that you are not good enough or you may lack confidence in your own abilities. You might have failed a test or exam in the past or performed badly or not been prepared for an exam and that caused you some trauma and fear that is replaying itself again now as exams approach.

You might find yourself extra anxious or procrastinating on getting stuck into your revision. We can look at what blocks might be lurking beneath the surface and remove these, so you forge ahead and get those results you so deserve.

Summary of Part One

What I would like you to take away from Part One is how complex the number and array of factors are that can be at play in how prone we are to stress and anxiety generally and how the pressure of exams increases that. I invite you to take those concepts that work for you and discard those that do not resonate.

These factors, if present, will each add to the load on your nervous system. Think of the snowball gathering more snow as it goes down a hill and that the point where everything spills over will be more quickly reached. Exams could well be that tipping point on an already stressed, exhausted nervous system. The more depleted we are the more easily overwhelmed we can become and the harder it is for us to be in that *safe and social* healing zone. The overload can be a gradual build up or it can be a more sudden onset with one thing being 'the straw that broke the camel's back', that quaint saying that we have to describe a massive sudden reaction or breakdown due to the cumulative effect of events.

I hope this section has helped you to understand and be more aware of why you might act or react to stress and why your exam anxiety is heightened. In Part Two you will find strategies and tools to find relief.

Part Two:
Solutions

Introduction

We are all individuals. What might work for one person might not work for you or might not resonate. All I ask is that you explore this section with an open mind, a growth mindset and from a place of curiosity.

Some of these tools and tips are simple to implement and others may take practice and perseverance. This leads me nicely on to the 5Ps.

The 5 Ps

As you engage with this material, please bear in mind the 5 Ps: *Patience, Practice, Perseverance, Persistence* and *Presence* (being fully present). Some of these tools will be quick wins you can implement immediately. Others may require more effort to try out and their benefits will come with consistency and practice.

It can take at least twenty-one days for a new neural pathway to be built and for a new activity or way of thinking to become a habit. We need to literally retrain and reprogramme our brains every day for at least this period of time.

Exam Preparation and Revision

In the lead up to exams, two more Ps here are crucial: *planning* and *preparation*. Have you ever heard the phrase 'By failing to prepare you are preparing to fail'? If you are prepared, this goes a long way toward helping you feel much more confident about the exams. And it can help decrease your anxiety.

Now I know some individuals (like my son) leave everything to the last minute. Whilst others, like my nephew, start planning and revising for exams an entire year ahead. What we are ideally aiming for is somewhere in between.

Think back to the Personality Types we looked at in Part One – the Type A and B, and the *Helper, Achiever, Controller, Perfectionist, Anxiety* behaviour patterns.

If you know you are a *perfectionist*, then you may need to build in some extra time but remember not to spend too long or to focus on one topic and to keep to the revision plan, so all topics are covered. And yes, I would say a revision plan is crucial for most people. Just the act of pulling one together will help you feel more at ease and in control.

With the *achiever*, think about your realistic expectations. Maybe have some contingency plans in place so if you don't get your first choice or get the grades you want there is a Plan B that ticks most of the boxes, even if it's not the obvious first choice.

I am a great believer that sometimes we can be set on a certain path we are planning to take but the universe has other ideas for us. I have had situations where I have been disappointed when I have not gotten what I wanted, such as a job, but ended up with a much better option a month or so later!

So, this was a big lesson for me and with hindsight I found that, when seemingly bad or unwelcome things happen to us, it could be for our highest good in the long run.

Remember that, whilst these exams are important, in the bigger context of our life they are not. There are plenty of examples where individuals have not done well in their exams but have gone on to have very successful and fulfilled lives: Simon Cowell left school with just two O levels; Lord Alan Sugar dropped out of school at age sixteen; Deborah Meaden dropped out of her A levels and studied business at Brighton Technical College; Richard Branson left school at sixteen; Stephen Spielberg was rejected by the University of Southern California Theatre, Film and TV but it didn't stop him from becoming one of the most prominent and successful film producers of all time. Now, I am not saying exams do not matter; I am merely making the point that if you don't do as well as you would like, it is not the end of the world.

Remember, too, that whilst the lead up to exams and the exams themselves may seem never ending, they will come to an end. Keeping in mind the phrase 'This too shall pass' can be helpful to remind us of this when we are going through a challenging time

Revision – Some Quick Tips

Sometimes it can seem an insurmountable task to get through everything, but I always remember this analogy: How do you eat an elephant? Whilst I do not recommend eating one at all, you would not attempt to eat it all in one go. You would break it down into small bite-sized pieces and you keep going. Consistency and a regular routine are key.

I am not going to go into this in too much detail as there are plenty of great resources out there but below are my top tips.

- Create a Revision Plan. Find a good template or use a diary – whatever works for you – and personalise it. There are loads that you can customise for your needs.

- Put in all your social activities and time for exercise too so you have everything in one place.

- If you know you work better in the morning, then schedule more sessions then. If you work better after school build your timetable around that.

- If you want a complete break on one day, maybe a Saturday, make sure you block that out.

- You might want to focus first on the subjects you like best but make sure you give yourself time to look at the subjects and topics you are not so keen to tackle. Break it down into bite-sized chunks, so it doesn't seem overwhelming.

- Think about how you learn. If you are visual, mind maps or images and drawings can come in handy. You might want to use colour codes. If you learn better by listening, then maybe record your notes so you can play them back to yourself. If you are a kinesthetic learner, you might make up games to help recall information.

- Consolidating all your notes into a revision book, or the key points for each topic onto an A4 page or flashcards, can be great to check you have covered and understood all the topics and to check for gaps in information. They are great to use as reminders/prompts of key information that you can quickly recap closer to the exam.

- Ensure you build in regular breaks when you revise. It's especially important not to be online for too long without a break. Research shows that your brain can only take in so much information. So, revise **SMARTER** not harder. And do what works for you. You might do an hour then take a break. If you find that is too long to concentrate and focus, break down study slots into twenty- or thirty-minute sessions.

- Make your breaks count and do something that you enjoy. It might be making yourself a drink, taking the dog out for a walk or doing twenty star-jumps. It might be helpful to think about what you will do in these breaks in advance to gain the most from them. Be disciplined about sticking to your timetable. And if it isn't working for you, then do not be afraid to adjust it.

- Test your knowledge with regular practice exam papers or multiple-choice questions and set yourself a timer to do these in the time allowed for the exam. Passing an exam is about knowledge, yes, but it is also about time management and organisation, which is a skill that comes with practice.

- Work in a quiet space where you are not going to get distracted or interrupted. Leave your phone in another room, so you can focus completely for the time set aside and you are not tempted to look at the latest alert that has come in. It used to be thought that multi-tasking was efficient but more recent research has shown that actually it isn't. Our minds flit between one task and another and this can take more energy and time than simply focusing on one thing before moving on to the next.

- Build in some time for setbacks, or for things not always going according to plan – a friend turning up unexpectedly, for example, or an appointment. This will give you a buffer.

- Little and often and consistency are key. Keep going. Remember that eating an elephant can take time and persistence!! Or, if you prefer, think of an artist chipping away at an ice block to make an ice sculpture. Each chip is a step closer to the work of art! It may seem a mammoth task and then suddenly it comes together.

- Build in nice treats and rewards for yourself. That might be watching a film or a favourite episode of a boxset, an online game with friends or taking the dog out for a walk. A nice treat for the dog too!

- At the end of the day remind yourself what you have achieved. Congratulate yourself on what you have done rather than focusing on what you still have ahead of you, or any setback.

- You might want to consider having a Done list where you tick off all the things you have covered. This can be very motivational in seeing what you have covered even if your To Do list is still seemingly very long and a bit overwhelming! If you have an *achiever* or *controller* behaviour pattern this might help you.

- Remember also that if it does get tough, acknowledge your feelings if you are getting a bit bogged down. Keep in mind, however, that our feelings do not equate to facts and try not to sink into a feeling of 'I can't do this', 'this is too hard', or 'I am never going to get there'. You will! Do not let it knock your confidence. Think about a tough time you have been through before and realise that you got through it. It can be helpful to look at what got you through that challenging time and draw on those strengths now too.

- Sometimes we can be extremely hard on ourselves with our self-talk and judgement so talk and act as if you are your own best friend or cheerleader. If a friend came to you putting themselves down you would not agree with them; you'd point out all the good things and boost their confidence, wouldn't you? Be that person to yourself. You can and should be your own best friend.

- There is no such word as failure in my vocabulary and I suggest you ban it from yours. Replace it with another F word – feedback! Much more positive and something we can grow and learn from.

- Remember you are not alone. It might seem like it, as you are settling down to study, but there are thousands of others in the same situation and probably feeling very much like you are.

- Remember exams take up a very small portion of your life, even though at the time it doesn't seem like it!

- You may like to revise with a friend to test each other. Or set up a study group of a few of you looking at a topic at the same time. You might want to build in time when you check in with each other, perhaps on WhatsApp or Snapchat or whatever you use. Share how it is going and share anything you are struggling with. This could be done online or in person. Make it social and inject fun into it, where you can.

- Talk to someone if you are struggling, a parent or a trusted adult, a friend, a teacher or your doctor/GP. Expressing and sharing how you are feeling can be such a relief. That adage is very true even though it may seem a bit cliched – a *problem shared is often a problem halved*. If you are in need of more immediate support in a particular moment then Childline is there for you twenty-four hours, seven days a week: https://www.childline.org.uk.

Parents (if they are around and are able to) can play a great role in the following:
- Helping put exam results in context.
- Reassuring students about expectations and being realistic/taking the pressure off.
- Helping students complete/review their revision timetable if appropriate.
- Keeping students not only motivated but also accountable to the timetable.

- Making sure regular breaks are taken.
- Supporting with drinks and mini snacks.
- Checking in on how things are going, gently nudging and encouraging where necessary.
- And on the more practical side, I have spent many an hour going on a walk with my son or during a car journey testing him on his latest topic. It has been helpful in identifying any gaps in his understanding and building confidence in what he has managed to retain. And it has made me feel I am doing something useful to help the cause.

Mindset and Change the Way You Think & Feel Tools

Being a clinical hypnotherapist I must mention the power of *mindset*. For me mindset is key. We have already discussed that the subconscious programming of our minds is far more powerful than our conscious logical brain. In fact, and this may surprise you, your thoughts are actually so powerful that they influence your reality.

Feeding positive thoughts and suggestions into your subconscious will, over time, build a more positive optimistic mental attitude.

Your mind will come to accept these as your reality. It cannot tell the difference between the imagined and the real.

If you think a goal is beyond you, then subconsciously you are unlikely to put the effort in to achieve it. Whereas, if you believe you can get there this opens a universe of possibilities for success. If you believe and think you can, you will! Simple as that! This is the concept of *neuroplasticity*, the brain's capability to grow and change in response to our experiences and learning. The brain can make new connections between neurons, re-organise existing ones and grow new cells. We have control over how we think and, therefore, our reality.

How do we reprogramme our brain? Well, there are two main elements you need: *repetition* and *consistency*.

There are several ways we can do this. My favourite way is using hypnosis as I genuinely believe it is one of the most powerful tools we have at our disposal.

Hypnosis

Hypnosis has been much misunderstood. People think immediately of stage hypnosis where an audience member is asked up on stage and hypnotised to act in silly ways – to cluck like a chicken, etc. That is an entertaining party trick, but it is not what I am talking about. What I am referring to is the trance-like state of focus and concentration that we are all in as we are about to fall asleep or upon first waking in the morning. This is a similar state to being completely absorbed in a book, movie, music or even one's own thoughts or when we are meditating. In this state of flow, we are in a Theta brainwave.

This heightened state of relaxation just distracts the conscious mind, allowing us to turn attention inward and access the subconscious. In this state, we can make changes or regain control in areas of life, even productively handling situations that have been causing fear, anxiety or blocking you, so you can reach your goals.

For many of my clients, I do this on a one-on-one basis, tailored to my exact client needs, but hypnosis can be done in a group or via a recording, through a guided meditation. Once a deep enough state is reached suggestions are made that the subconscious takes on board.

These can be along the lines of: *You are finding it easy to revise. You are taking in everything you read. You retain the information easily and can recall it effortlessly. You are relaxed and confident about the exams and looking forward to showing what you know.*

The key is *repetition* and using the *present tense*. The brain cannot tell the difference between the real and the imagined, so we instil these suggestions into the subconscious mind where they take root and become reality. We are basically training the brain to think in a different way, creating a new neural pathway. It takes at least twenty-one days, as I have said before, for a new neural pathway or habit to form, so I recommend that recordings are listened to at least every night for that time – ideally longer.

Affirmations

Affirmations are statements, phrases or suggestions that you give to yourself. And they work on the same basis as explored above. As you give yourself these suggestions, they programme the subconscious mind and build that positive mindset. It is like planting seeds – in time they grow and can start to draw in the positive opportunities and your goals towards you.

One study showed students who used affirmations at the start of the school term performed better than their peers who didn't use affirmations.

Starting with Affirmations

A great way to start is to sit down and write down all your fears and worries and then turn them into positive affirmations. For example:

Negative Thought	Positive Affirmation
I can't do this.	I can do this. I am doing this. I am going to do my best/I am doing my best.
I can't remember this topic.	My brain recalls this topic easily.

Affirmations need to be in the *positive* and *present* tense. The 'I AM' format works well.

Below are some examples of affirmations you might like to use.

Self-belief
- I believe in myself.
- I am worthy of good exam results.
- I deserve to do well.
- I am achieving my goals.
- I can have the results I want.
- I choose to focus on all the positives in my life.
- Things always work out for me.
- I am doing my best.
- I am proud of what I have done/achieved.

Confidence
- My confidence grows more and more every day.
- I am taking revision/exams in my stride.
- I am a talented and hard-working student.
- I can do this/I am doing this.
- I am nailing this/I have got this!
- I am doing the best I can.
- I approve of myself.

Memory/Learning
- I know everything I need to know for this exam.
- I always remember what I've learned.
- I'm a quick learner.
- I have a perfect/good memory.
- I recall facts and information easily.
- I have plenty of time and resources available to me.
- Revision and exams come easy to me.
- I approach my revision/every test or exam with confidence and determination.
- I am organized and disciplined in my studies.
- My mind is a sponge and absorbs everything I read and see.
- I see the exam as an opportunity to share all I know.

Anxiety
- I am feeling calm/I am calm.
- I am feeling in control/I am in control.
- Inside, I am calm.
- I breathe, I am collected, and I am calm.
- Nothing can disturb my peacefulness.
- My anxiety becomes less and less every day.
- My anxiety doesn't control my life. I do.

- I let go/release fear/doubt/anxiety/worry/tension/negative thinking.
- I choose only to think good thoughts.
- I am safe.
- I am okay.
- Everything is good in my world.
- I have come so far.
- I am proud of me.
- Things are getting better and easier.
- I determine how I feel, and I am choosing to feel safe/calm/good.
- This too shall pass.
- This is just one moment in my life.
- I breathe and take it one breath at a time.
- I give/allow myself space.
- I am kind to myself.

Have a go at pulling together your own!

Note: It is important you use the language and words that resonate with you. You also need to feel that your affirmations are within your reach and attainable. Research has shown that if you pick something that is too ambitious or too much of a stretch too soon, it can be de-motivating. Better to start small and work up.

How to use affirmations

Say them aloud to yourself as often as you can. There is a great power in saying them aloud. Really say them with intention and feeling. Mentally repeat them too. I like to write the ones I am working on at any time on Post-It Notes and dot them around the house and put them on mirrors in the bathroom too. So, every time I clean my teeth, I see them and say them to myself. That way I know that I am saying them at least twice a day! Put them on your walls or your desk too if you like. Record them on your phone and play them back or turn them into a song. Or you can write them in a journal. The more different ways of using them and all the senses the better.

It is a great exercise to catch yourself if you think something negative. Then turn it into a positive 'I AM' statement. For example, turn 'I can't do this' into 'I can and I am doing this, I'm working hard and I am getting there'.

You do need to practice them *daily* to get the most from them. Remember the 5 Ps (Practice, Persistence, Patience, Perseverance,

Presence). Remember the twenty-one days to form a habit/belief, and keep going.

I also recommend the use of affirmations in parallel with using a hypnosis recording. The subconscious cannot help but respond.

ANTS Way of Thinking Exercise

ANTs stands for Automatic Negative Thoughts. ANTs are toxic thoughts that are not helpful to us.

Our thinking and our thoughts influence our mood, behaviour and the way we experience the world. If you think the world is an unfriendly place, then that is what you will experience. Awareness allows us space to observe and to make adjustments. Just do this with curiosity and no judgement.

If you are not sure of your tendencies, ask a family member or trusted friend which ones they notice you slip into.

Make a real effort for a week to really focus on these and catch yourself if you start to fall into one of these tendencies. Then, come back and

Type of ANT	More detailed explanation	How often do you fall into the pattern? *Rarely, Sometimes, Often*	What could you do differently? Fill in the boxes to help you shift. *(I've done the first one for you!)*
All or nothing thinking	Also known as black and white thinking		Is there a different view I haven't considered? Is there a middle way I have not thought about?
"Always" thinking	Using words like *always, never, no one, everyone, every time, everything*		
Focusing on the Negative	Selectively seeing the bad or negative in a situation and disregarding any of the good		
Fortune Telling	Jumping to and predicting the worst case scenario/outcome		
Mind Reading	Believing you know what someone else is thinking even though she or he hasn't told you		
Believing your Feelings	You don't question them, just take them as fact or truth, even when there is no evidence to support how you feel		
Guilt Beating	Using words like *should, must, have to, ought to*		
Labelling	Calling yourself or another a derogatory name and not seeing the situation clearly		
Blaming	Not taking responsibility for your actions, i.e., it is someone else's fault. (You abdicate your power to make change when you do this.)		

*Go to https://amity-health.com/teens-book/ to download this worksheet see if any of those you have marked above as 'Often' have shifted to either 'Sometimes' or 'Rarely'.

You might find the STOP process a little further on can help you break some of these habits too.

Change Your Language Change Your Mind Exercise

It really is true that if you start to look at your language and the words you use, you really can shift things to a more positive perspective.

This is all about being kinder to yourself, too, being your own best friend.

Here are some words to look out for and some alternatives for you to try. Again, the more you do this the easier it will become.

Should/need to/ought to/have to:
- I *should* go and do my revision.
- I *should* go and exercise.
- I *should* eat healthily.

Tune into how this sounds as you say it. How does it feel in your body? When I say it, I sense a real feeling of reluctance. I hear 'This is a chore and effort; I really don't want to do this'. Does it feel heavy and as if your mind and body are resisting it? It feels like it comes from a place of 'I really don't want to' and it almost feels like a punishment. This isn't going to put you in the right frame of mind to start off with. It feels disempowering.

Whereas, when you slightly change the language to 'I *choose*' or 'I *get to*', see how that feels. To me it feels much more empowering, much more positive. You are in control.

- I *choose* to go and do my revision.
- I *choose* to go and exercise.
- I *choose* to eat healthily.

Come up with your own list of *I shoulds* and switch them to *I choose* or *I get to:*

I should/need to/ ought to/have to	I choose to/I get to
I should/need to/ ought to/have to	
I should/need to/ ought to/have to	
I should/need to/ ought to/have to	

*Go to https://amity-health.com/teens-book/ to download this worksheet

How can this help during exams? Using 'I choose to' or 'I get to' rather than 'I have to' gives you back a feeling of choice and control and feels like a positive way forward.

How do you begin your day?

Our first thoughts in the morning on waking can really set the tone for the day ahead. Do you open your eyes and groan 'here we go again, another day to get through'? During stressful periods of time waking each day can feel heavy. You might feel dread at having to do things you might not want to, like revision or even an exam. That feeling will just accompany you through the day, and we don't want that do we?

So, try this instead. Before you even open your eyes, spend a few moments being grateful for your bed, your room and all the good things in your life. And remember those affirmations? You might like to go through a few of those in your mind, affirming that everything is going to go well for you. I challenge you to do this for a week and see the difference it makes in how you feel. I hope you will find it so beneficial that it will start to become part of your daily routine. It only takes seconds.

How can this help during exams? It can set a positive tone for your day ahead and remind you that making revision and exams are just a part of your life, not your whole life.

Having a regular 'Worry Time'

If you do feel some worry, then why not spend five or so minutes writing all of those worries out on paper or in a journal? (We talk more about using a journal in section *Journaling & Automatic or Free Writing*). Sometimes just getting things out of your head and onto paper can help clear the mind.

Just ask yourself 'What am I worried about?' List all your concerns and worries on one side of the page. Then go back and review them and see if they are true worries or if you can do something about them. You can then put in a potential plan of what you will do and when, or something that will make you feel better about the situation.

If during the day another worry surfaces you might then say to yourself 'I'll put that aside until my worry time'. Having a regular worry time might be a routine that you want to adopt going forwards so worries do not spill into every part of your day. And when one does you know you can pull together a plan to deal with it.

Below are a couple of tools you might find helpful as you think of your worries: the *Catch it/Check it/Change it* and *Think Tool*.

Catch it/Check it/Change it

I find this a helpful way of remembering how the above process could work.

1. Capture your thoughts (Catch it).

2. Ask yourself if they are actually true worries (Check it).

3. Look at how you might change them (Change it).

THINK Tool

T	It is true?
H	Is it helpful?
I	Is it inspiring?
N	Is it necessary?
K	Is it kind to me?

If the answer to these is no, then make a shift to change it into something more positive and affirming.

How can this help during exams? It can help you empty out all of your worries before you start your day and hopefully ease some of them so you engage more fully in the day ahead without distraction.

Worst Case Scenario and What if? Tool

I love these two tools. One of my friends taught these to me many years ago. It was the way she looked at life. If I was a bit down or worried about something she'd say to me 'What is the worst that can happen?' According to her, the worst thing for her would be to die, so she'd say to me 'You are not going to die, are you? So what are you worried about then?' It really did make me think she had a point and helped to put things in perspective for me.

So, what is the worst that can happen? You don't get your grades to go to the school/college or university of your choice?

So, *what if*, then?

You do a different course somewhere else. *What if* that happens?

You go out to work. *What if* that happens?

You retake your exams. *What if* that happens?

Using the *What if?* question, you peel down the layers of all the different possibilities. This can diffuse the fear and make the scary not so scary after all.

Think of a young child in bed at night in the dark convinced there is a monster under the bed. The only real way to prove that there is actually no monster is to look under the bed and see that there is nothing there. So we use the same concept with the *What if* tool and we look the worst case scenario in the eye.

More times than not, the thing that was looming so big and large is no longer quite such a big deal. We may not want any of these outcomes but;

1. The world has not come to an end, to my friend's point, and;

2. Unexpected situations occur in life that were not in our plans but many times we may look back and see in hindsight that actually they have led us to something that was perhaps a better option for us. It just wasn't obvious or we just hadn't seen it at the time.

Try using the *What if* tool to look at the potential positives of the situation you are facing too. Some examples are below of how you could use this.

- What if today is a really great day?
- What if things go better than I think?
- What if everything works out for me?
- What if something good comes from this?
- What if I learn and grow from this?

Can you see how this invites in the possibility (and therefore the energy) of something more positive?

How can this help during exams? It can help you face your deepest worries and to realise that even if this were to happen, there are always options and solutions available to you and it can shift the energy into the positive.

Reframing Exercise

If you find yourself slipping into negative thinking ask 'Are these thoughts/beliefs really true?' Have a go at how you might be able to reframe the negative phrases below in a more positive way. (I have done the first couple for you.)

Remember when we talked about mindset and energy? If we think or say something we are giving it energy, and the possiblity of it becoming a reality, so, by turning it into a positive reframe we are literally shifting it into something more positive. I have a whole section on energy and vibration below. Check it out. You might like to use these as affirmations when you are finished.

Negative	Positive Reframe
I am going to fail	*You don't know that, so change this to something along the lines of:* I am going to do my best. *How much better does that feel? Test both in your body and 'feel' the difference.*
My nerves are going to get the better of me	I have done everything I can. Nerves are natural and I have lots of tools and tips to keep them at bay.
Everyone else has done more revision than I have	
I can't seem to take anything in or remember anything	
I am awful at exams	
I am not going to remember anything in the exam	
I am not going to get the grades I want or need	
I am going to let myself and everyone else down	
These exams are the be all and end all	

*Go to https://amity-health.com/teens-book/ to download this worksheet

How can this help during exams? It can quickly shift you out of negative into a more positive way of thinking.

Five Step Anxiety Release Exercise

Grab a pen and paper and write down the answers to these questions.

1. What is one thing I am anxious about today?

2. What is one thing I could do to prevent or prepare for it?

3. What is one reason it probably isn't going to be as bad as I think it is?

4. What is one reason I know I could probably handle it?

5. What is one possible upside of the situation?

The STOP Process

This is a tool that I often use with my clients. It does take practice and it's based on recognising patterns of behaviour. One of my favourite phrases I use with my clients is 'If you can SEE it, you can SHIFT it' (for short, See it and Shift it). This means that if you are aware of a pattern of behaviour you can make a conscious choice to not go into that pattern and react differently. It puts you in control.

It is a simple tool that you can use for exam anxiety, but it can also be used much more widely to help break negative patterns, thoughts or behaviours. You can use it when you start to fall into negative thinking or notice your anxiety is being triggered. You can even use it for when you are about to reach for that bar of chocolate or packet of crisps that you know you don't really want or need.

The steps are as follows:
1. Notice or recognise the pattern and behaviour you are falling into.

2. Say aloud to yourself 'STOP'. If you can, use hand gestures too, putting both hands up as if to gesture to someone else to stop. If you are with people and it isn't appropriate to say stop out loud, say it to yourself mentally or very quietly.

3. Notice at this point that *you* have a *choice*. You are in control. You can decide whether to continue down this cycle or you can choose differently. Shift your attention to your body by shaking or wriggling your toes and feet, or distract yourself by doing something else (taking a shower, listening to music).

4. Congratulate yourself on choosing differently. This helps you feel like you have achieved something, a form of positive reinforcement that makes you more likely to do this again.

This process does take practice, perseverance, and persistence. If you try it and it doesn't work, please keep going with it. Do not give up because I promise you that you are training yourself to *respond* (not *react*) in a different way and that does take time. The more you do this the more natural it will become and, before long, you'll find you do this automatically.

The STOP process just gives you a chance to take a step back and gives you that breathing space to just ask yourself 'Do I really want this?' and to recognise 'I have a choice about how I react and respond'.

I recommend putting the STOP process on some Post-It Notes and dotting them around your home or your bedroom as a reminder.

How can this help during exams? It can stop you spiralling into a negative pattern of thought or actions and reiterates that you are in control of your thoughts and actions.

Situation – Feeling – Response Model

Similarly, the *Situation – Feeling – Response* model can also be useful to recognise what your stress and anxiety triggers might be.

Remember in *Stress Overload* in Part One when we looked at the two different factors that can add to our stress – external and internal stressors? The model works in this way:

Situation/Trigger – Becoming aware of an event or circumstance that triggers you.

Feeling – What emotional feeling/felt sense in

the body does this evoke?

Response – How you tend to respond.

Example:
Situation/Trigger – A friend is talking about how much revision they have done.

Feeling – This makes you feel nervous. You can feel the fear rising and possibly even panic that you haven't done enough. Your breathing might become a bit shallow; you might experience a heavy, sick feeling in the pit of your stomach.

Response – You beat yourself up for not doing more. This may spark you to go into 'revision overdrive' in a panic, or it may deflate you so you feel it isn't worth trying as you won't ever catch up.

Once you know what your pattern is you can notice it and then use the STOP process above. Choose to not fall into that pattern and use that best friend inner voice to say to yourself, 'It is fine. I am doing the best I can. I have worked hard, and I am not going into that rabbit hole of comparison as everyone is different. I am going to just concentrate on me.'

See how this works? See it and shift it. Change your thinking, change your mind and your state.

Just be curious about your triggers and responses. No judgment or blame, just notice the feelings as they come up, with interest.

Emotions and Feelings

Clients often ask what the difference is between an *emotion* and a *feeling*. These two terms are sometimes used interchangeably. However, an emotion for me usually comes before a feeling. An emotion is literally *energy in motion*. I think of emotions as responsible for what we are feeling, and we tend to experience those feelings in our physical body.

So, to clarify here is a simplified chain of events as I understand it; our beliefs and thoughts lead to an emotion that leads to a feeling in our body, creating our physical reality.

There is a school of thought that believes there are only two main emotions – *love* and *fear* – and the rest of our emotions are branches of one or the other of these. (See a list of example emotions below.) You are either in the energy of love or fear – you cannot be in both at once. So, when it comes to anxiety, we are at the fear end of the spectrum. The aim is to bring you back into love (remember safe and social mode) and, where there is no fear, no anxiety or worry. Hence, I recommend you do things that bring you love and joy as often as you can, at least once, if not more, a day, as it is a great tool to get out of a fear/worry state.

Leading on from this, did you know that there is a theory that the energy or frequency of emotions can be measured in hertz?

Lower emotions sit at the bottom of the scale, at 20 hertz and above:

Shame	20 Hz
Guilt	30 Hz
Apathy	59 Hz
Fear	100 Hz
Anger	150 Hz

Higher emotions sit at the top of the scale, at 300 hertz and above:

Courage	200 Hz
Acceptance	350 Hz
Love	500 Hz
Joy	540 Hz
Peace	600 Hz

The benefit of such a scale is being able to see where you are at, at any given time, especially if you are spending prolonged periods of time at the bottom. It can give us the impetus to raise our energy to get ourselves to a higher frequency. Just by asking ourselves 'what do I need to do to bring more joy or love into my life?' can be helpful. It is not expected that we can go from shame to acceptance just like that, but we can perhaps choose to aim for an emotion a little higher up the scale and work towards that.

Some Example Emotions

You might like to use this list (not exhaustive, just to help you work out what you are feeling). I have categorised them into low and high energy. High energy feels intense and low energy less intense. As you read the words focus on how each of them feels in your body. The more you do this the more able you will be to recognise what you are feeling in your body.

Fear/Anxiety/Worry:

Negative High Energy	Terrified, petrified, despairing, angry, outraged, triggered, explosive, anxious, worried, frustrated, anguished, livid, enraged, repulsed, rejected, peeved, outraged, repulsed, upset, hopeless
Negative Low Energy	Sad, depressed, apathetic, wounded, numb, grief, glum, isolated, defensive, disappointed, fatigued, tired, sullen, uneasy, heavy, spent, low, drained, resentful

Love/Joy:

Positive High Energy	Joyful, happy, elated, vibrant, enthusiastic, invigorated, cheerful, lively inspired, amazed, excited, buzzing, exuberant, vital, ecstatic, fantastic, blissful, grateful
Positive Low Energy	Peaceful, calm, restful, serene, tranquil, in control, comfortable, at ease, mellow, satisfied, positive, tolerant, accepting, hopeful, balanced, content, fulfilled

It makes sense to be operating at the highest frequency we can. Why? Because energy attracts energy and if we are in that higher vibration we will attract higher energy. When we are in the lower vibration, we find it harder to deal with more challenging situations and circumstances. We ideally want to be in the energy of when everything just seems to slot into place and flows. In essence and in practice, this means trying to live most of our time in those higher emotions of joy and happiness, gratitude and peace and calm. We cannot be there, as we have said, all the time. However, if you find yourself spending too long in the lower emotions of fear, worry and frustration, then there are various tools you can use to shift your energy to a higher frequency/vibration. We will look at these in more detail in section *Sound Therapy/Raising Our Vibration Tool*.

Sitting with our Emotions and Feelings

So many of us are frightened of feeling or expressing our emotions, especially what I call the darker, low energy ones, but, if that is what we are feeling, we need to honour them – the fear, sadness, shame, guilt and despair.

It is part of being human that we have a full spectrum of emotions to experience. We live in a world of duality. We do not have day without night, light without darkness. We would not know we were happy if we didn't have sadness and other low frequency emotions.

What I do know is that we tend to stuff down the more negative emotions, as we feel that if we go there, we might get stuck. It really helped me when I learned that emotions come and go.

Emotion = Energy in Motion

Each emotion usually only lasts for ninety seconds before another one comes along. Energy in motion, remember. So, if we sit with the emotion, as difficult as it may seem, it will usually dissipate. I like to think of clouds that come and go on a breezy day. They are always changing and reforming.

I love this quote by Tara Brach, American psychologist and author: 'All any feeling wants is to be welcomed with tenderness. It wants room to unfold. It wants to relax and tell its story.'

Feelings are just your body trying to communicate with you, giving you real-time feedback. If we do not acknowledge our emotions or process them and, instead, we stuff them down or ignore them, they can cause blockages, adding to that stress load we talked about in section *Stress Overload* in Part One. This can lead to energy depletion and even physical illness.

My recommendation is, if you can, to sit with the emotion, even if it feels hard. Acknowledge it, being curious about how it is showing up in your body. Does it feel heavy? Achy? Light? Tingly? Warm? Cold?

Try this exercise and see how you get on. The more you do this the more natural it will become.

Sitting with Negative Emotions – BACK Exercise

B	Breathe	Pause and acknowledge and name the emotion if you can, e.g., I am feeling anger/fear.
A	Allow	Give yourself permission to feel. Meet the emotion here without judgement, just curiosity. 'I am feeling x.' Ask 'How can I soften my resistance to this and be present with what is here?'
C	Connect	Connect with your body. What am I feeling and where? Is it felt in your head, heart, stomach, etc? How does it feel there? Light, heavy, tight, tingly? Ask, 'What is this really about? What do I need most right now?' Do not worry if you don't get an answer. That is absolutely fine.
K	Kiss	Nurture that part of you. Say 'I hear you. I see you. You matter. Thank you for showing me.'

Remember that emotions shift and another one can come along. So if, as you are doing this exercise, you become aware of a different or deeper, more vulnerable, emotion coming up, just sit with that too.

If you'd like to explore further, then you can keep going.

1. When you get to what you think is the bottom emotion, ask yourself:

- What is really getting to me here?
- Is there an action I can take to resolve this? What would I normally do?
- Could I see this situation/emotion in a different way?
- Could I do something different?

2. Ask yourself 'How do I ideally want to feel?' Try to feel this ideal feeling in your body or imagine yourself feeling this. For example, if you want to feel relaxed or joyful, think of a time when you have felt that or something close to that. How did that feel in your body?

Do not worry if you find this hard to do at first. It takes time. You could always ask yourself 'How would that feel, if I **could** feel that? What might that feel like?' And use your imagination.

To end the exercise, you could close with saying to yourself out loud or in your head mentally 'I now choose to let go of all the negative emotions and to hold on to all the positive feelings I have tapped into.'

You might at this point like to capture in writing (or painting or drawing) what your takeaways of this exercise were. See sections *Automatic Writing* and *Intuitive Drawing/Painting* for details about how to do this.

How can this help during exams? Learning to listen to your emotions and process them and let them go means they don't get stuck and weigh you down. They can be released, lightening your load. And it can show you where you need to take some action to soothe or be kind to yourself too.

Sound Therapy/Raising Our Vibration Tool

Sound and music are the fastest and easiest ways to raise your mood and energy. Listening to your favourite music can be really helpful. My only caveat is that you listen to something that is upbeat to raise you up rather than something that is deep, slow and more soulful, as that will not have the same effect.

Also, check out music that operates at 852 hertz. Remember the Scale of Consciousness and vibration of emotions we explored in section *Emotions and Feelings*? This is believed to be a healing frequency of love and joy. You can find lots of music and mediations online that will raise and lift your spirits.

I love dancing and I know that even dancing around my kitchen for five minutes can do wonders for my emotional and physical energy. Movement of any kind can be great, but add music in and it can really help lift you.

If you have the chance to experience a sound healing bath with gongs or crystal Tibetan bowls (if offered in your local area), they can be a great way of relaxing and shifting energy. You can find recordings online for free otherwise. You lie down and listen to a practitioner play these bowls for thirty to sixty minutes. The vibration of the sound has been shown to release physical and emotional blocks in the body.

How can this help during exams? They can instantaneously lift your mood and reinvigorate you as well as relax you, depending on the type and frequency of music you choose.

Tools to Get Us Back into Safe and Social

In Part One, we explored how, when we are overstressed or in a chronic state of anxiety, we are in *fight, flight or freeze* mode. Our bodies need to get back into feeling *safe and social* to operate at our best. In this section we will look at tools to calm our nervous systems down and get us back into a feeling of safety and security in our bodies.

Mindfulness, Meditation and Breathwork

Mindfulness is just being more present. When we are in the present it is harder for us to worry and be anxious because we are just in that moment. Nothing from the past or fear about the future can come in. Remember we talked about dissociation in Part One as part of the Freeze state. Mindfulness is consciously being in the body and being present to how we are feeling (bringing in all our senses) and being aware of our surroundings. The concept is that we just focus on one moment at a time. This is a great tool to help manage anxiety.

'Living in the now is the truest path to happiness.'

—Ekhart Tolle

Try these simple exercises.

Piece of Fruit Mindfulness Exercise

1. Choose a piece of fruit you like to eat: apple, orange, banana or strawberry. You can even do this with a raisin, if you prefer.

2. Hold whatever you have chosen in your hand. Observe its weight, size and texture. What do you notice? How does it feel to you?

Tools to Get Us Back into Safe and Social

3. Bring the fruit up to your nose and take a deep breath in. How does it smell?

4. When you are ready, put a piece in your mouth and see how that feels and then take a bite and chew it very slowly. What does it taste like? As you are chewing it how does the texture change?

5. Finally, swallow the fruit and see how that feels.

Did you notice how much more you appreciated and savoured the experience rather than gulping it down without a thought?

Think about how this exercise can help us slow down and savour each moment of our lives. Even when times are challenging we can stop and be in the moment – it can really help us appreciate what is going on for us right now. Try to be more mindful in whatever you are doing. Really be fully present in that moment.

You also might find having a mindful shower can help shift a heavy mood. Really feel the water and focus on how it feels as it comes into contact with the different areas of your body. Try different temperatures. Turn the dial up hot and then turn it to cold and feel the invigorating water wash over you. Even when your body is resisting it can feel wonderfully refreshing. Try to stand under the cold for sixty to ninety seconds. The research is still in its early days but immersing in cold water is supposed to boost our immunity and, on an exam day, if you are feeling a bit groggy, it will get the blood flowing and wake you up – even if it is a bit of a shock to the system.

Here is a mindful exercise going inwards to really appreciate yourself and how you are feeling, and to help shift any heaviness or tension.

Hand on Heart and Hand on Tummy Quick Exercise

So quick and easy yet it can bring comfort in minutes.

1. Sit comfortably and take a deep breath in through the nose and out through the mouth.

2. Place one hand on your heart and the other on your tummy. Close your eyes.

3. Just sit for a moment. Breathe and feel your hand on your heart and tummy go up as you breathe in and go down as you breathe out. Just do this for a few breaths. Allow any thoughts you are having to just gently come and go. No need to give them any importance or to try to get rid of them. Just observe them.

You might want to just finish there, or you can go on to step 4:

4. Home in on any area where you feel or sense there is anxiety or tension. Then, just imagine, see or sense yourself breathing into that area. Send love, compassion and acceptance if that feels appropriate to you to do so. Some of my clients like to imagine pink, gold and white light filling up that area and the tightness or tension dissolving.

Meditation

I so often hear 'I can't do meditation; I can't sit still long enough to focus. It doesn't work for me'. I thought the same at first, as the term conjures up sitting cross-legged for long periods of time. It does not have to be that way as the simple exercise above shows. There are so many types of meditation – my favourite is just being out walking in the forest and being with my thoughts (see *Mindful Walking Meditation* below). I also love listening to light relaxing music. Find a method that works for you.

Connecting with our breath really brings us into the body and can calm down our nervous system.

Try an app – there are plenty of free online options. Some of my top choices are:

- Headspace.
- Calm.
- Buddhify.
- Insight Timer.
- Simple Habit.

And remember the 5 Ps. I encourage you to give meditation time. Start slowly – a few minutes at first – and build up. Don't give up if it doesn't work for you immediately.

How can this help during exams? It allows you to pause the anxiety, putting it in its place, and to witness and explore it with acceptance. It just is. It can prevent you from going into an automatic pattern of reacting, reacting, giving you relief and control.

Having a Happy or Safe Place

Think of a place, person or something that makes you feel safe or brings you joy. I often think of my lovely King Charles Cavalier, Rosie, snuggling up to me and it immediately brings a smile to my face and I can feel my heart open.

You might like to think of a time when you felt totally relaxed and happy. For me I am at my most relaxed out walking in the beautiful forest close to my home. Any time I feel I need a quick boost or need to feel safe and comforted I just use my imagination and picture myself there.

If you can't immediately think of a happy memory just use your imagination to think about how feeling safe and relaxed might feel to you and base the exercise on that.

Whatever memory or image you are tapping into, zoom into the scene to look at it in detail. Are you alone? With others? Where are you? Outside or inside? Immerse yourself as deeply as you can in the experience, as if you are experiencing it right then and there again.

In my example, I am aware of the sun shining through the trees, hearing the sounds of the birds and the peace and tranquillity. I can feel and sense the warmth of the sunshine on my skin, how the slight breeze feels against my exposed skin. I immediately feel safe and feel any tension or stress leaving my body. Even though I am not physically there right at that moment, my body relaxes as if it were. The brain cannot distinguish between the real and imaginary. In fact, I used this image successfully when I had my son. It kept me so calm and peaceful that I did not need any pain medication whatsoever.

Experiment with what image and scene works for you.

How can this help during exams? It can give you much-needed space and immediately transport you into feeling safe, lighter and more relaxed.

Breathwork

Usually when we are anxious or nervous our breathing becomes shallower. Consciously being aware of our breath, and slowing it down, can be one of the things that calms our nervous system instantaneously, bringing us back into *safe and social* mode.

I have given you a few examples below of breathing exercises to try out. There might be one you find more helpful and calming, or you might like to alternate between them.

Counting to 10

Sit quietly and observe your breath. As you breathe in count one and as you exhale count two. Continue counting until you reach 10. Repeat for as long as you need.

Box Breathing 4 by 4 Exercise

I like doing this while tracing my finger around a mobile phone or a book.

1. Trace you finger up the long left-hand side of your mobile phone and breathe in for a count of four.

2. Trace your finger along the top as you hold the breath for a count of four.

3. Trace your finger down the right-hand side of your phone as you exhale for a count of four.

4. Trace your finger along the bottom of the phone as you hold your breath for a count of four.

Repeat as many times as you need to, until you feel calmer.

4-7-8 (Relaxation) Breath

This can be done anywhere too.

1. Inhale quietly through your nose to a mental count of four.

2. Hold your breath for a count of seven.

3. Exhale completely through your mouth, making a whoosh sound to a count of eight.

This is one breath cycle. Now inhale again and repeat for a total of four cycles.

Spine Alignment Breath Exercise

1. Sit up straight, imagining you have a string pulling you up from the crown of your head and your spine aligning gently.

2. Close your eyes if you feel comfortable (otherwise just lower your gaze downwards).

3. Put one hand gently on your chest and the other on your abdomen.

4. Take a deep breath in through your nose as you count to four and feel your abdomen and chest expand outwards. (Your hand on your chest and abdomen will be pushed outwards.) Focus all your attention on the breath.

5. After inhaling for a count of four, slowly exhale for a count of six, letting all the air

release from your lungs. Your abdomen and chest will contract inwards. (The slower you exhale, the more you'll engage the sympathetic nervous system. This signals to your body it is okay.) Repeat three times (or longer if you need to).

6. You might like to end the exercise by saying to yourself 'I am okay/I am calm/I am safe/I have got this/I can do this' (whatever feels right for you).

You might like to adopt this exercise to do each morning before your day. And if you do, then feel free to add in a step 7: Setting an intention or goal for your day.

How can this help during exams? When we are anxious our breathing becomes shallow. Breathing exercises can help us breathe deeper and get a grip on our anxiety whilst calming our nervous system down. It also brings us back into our body if we find we are dissociating. It can give us the space to take back control.

Mini Stretch

We carry so much tension in our heads, necks, and shoulders. This very quick stretch can be done at any time to relieve tightness. It's great for doing at your desk whilst revising or it can be done discreetly enough, even in an exam.

1. Tilt your head forward and slowly turn it to the left then back to the right. You might like to then go round clockwise and then anticlockwise. Whatever feels comfortable to you. Do not overstretch.

2. Raise your eyebrows up and down a few times (loosening your facial muscles).

3. Gently press the tip of your tongue to the roof of your mouth (the jaw and mouth also hold a lot of tension).

4. Shrug your shoulders up and hold them up for a few seconds and then release them back down. Repeat a few times.

Smile

Now I hope this one will provoke a smile! It is so simple but believe me it works really well and there are studies to back this up. Smiling tricks your brain into thinking everything's okay, even if it's not. Even if you are not feeling in the mood to smile, simply moving your face and jaw muscles into a smile can shift your mood. 'Fake it till you make it.' Believe me, it works.

Laugh

Have you heard of Laughter Yoga? It works in the same way as smiling does. As with smiling, if you do not feel like it, keep going, fake it and before you know it the energy of laughter will just overtake you. Laughter is infectious and a great release of tension, lowering stress hormones. Maybe try it with a group of friends and you will be amazed at how the laughter, after starting off quite forced, becomes very natural and infectious (in a good way).

How can this help during exams? It can quickly shift your energy and mood.

Give Yourself a Hug!

When we are upset our loved ones give us a hug. Or, if others are sad our natural inclination is to reach out and put an arm around them. We realised how much this contact with other humans is necessary during COVID when we couldn't touch and had to keep our distance.

So why not give *yourself* a hug or a cuddle when you need it most? This can be very self-soothing. Studies show that touch (even our own) releases oxytocin and serotonin, both of which lower our cortisol stress levels. If a hug feels a step too far and a bit strange just start off by stroking your arms in a downward direction with just the right amount of touch and pressure for you. You might want to rock back and forth too if that also feels comforting. Although a hug won't eradicate anxiety it can help relieve tension.

Peace Begins with Me

I learnt this technique from Gabrielle Bernstein, American motivational speaker and author. I teach it to lots of my clients of all ages. It can be done in seconds and can be very discreet.

Whenever I feel anxious or stressed, I simply tap my thumb on each of my fingers in turn and say the words.

Peace – as I touch the first finger.
Begins – as I touch the middle finger.
With – as I touch the ring finger.
Me – as I touch the little finger.

You can do this with both hands at once if you like.

Do it as many times as you need. You do not even need to say the words out loud. Just say it in your head, especially if you are around people and you do not want to draw attention to yourself.

It is remarkably grounding. The magic of it is in saying the words but also activating the acupressure points on each finger, which is believed can help energy flow and shift. How cool is that?

EFT/Emotional Freedom Technique (also known as Tapping)

As an EFT Practitioner, I highly recommend this technique. It is a great tool for clearing emotional distress and for pain relief. Based on Chinese medicine, it is similar to acupuncture (without the needles, you will be pleased to hear!). All you do is tap your fingers on various meridian points in the body. Very simply, meridian points are areas of the body that energy flows through. When these get blocked, we can get stuck or ill. By tapping on them you release the energy and allow it to flow again.

This tapping, combined with talking and expressing very honestly what you are feeling in the moment, allows you to release negative tension, energy and pain and gain relief. It changes your response to an event or experience.

The Tapping Meridian Points

Studies have shown EFT to be highly effective in treating stress and PTSD. A group of war veterans had EFT coaching sessions and, within a month, they had significantly reduced their psychological stress compared to those having standard care. And more than 50% no longer were considered to have PTSD.

A recent study (August 2023) by Dr Peta Stapleton found that Tapping held its own against treatments such as CBT (Cognitive

Teens Easing Exam Nerves

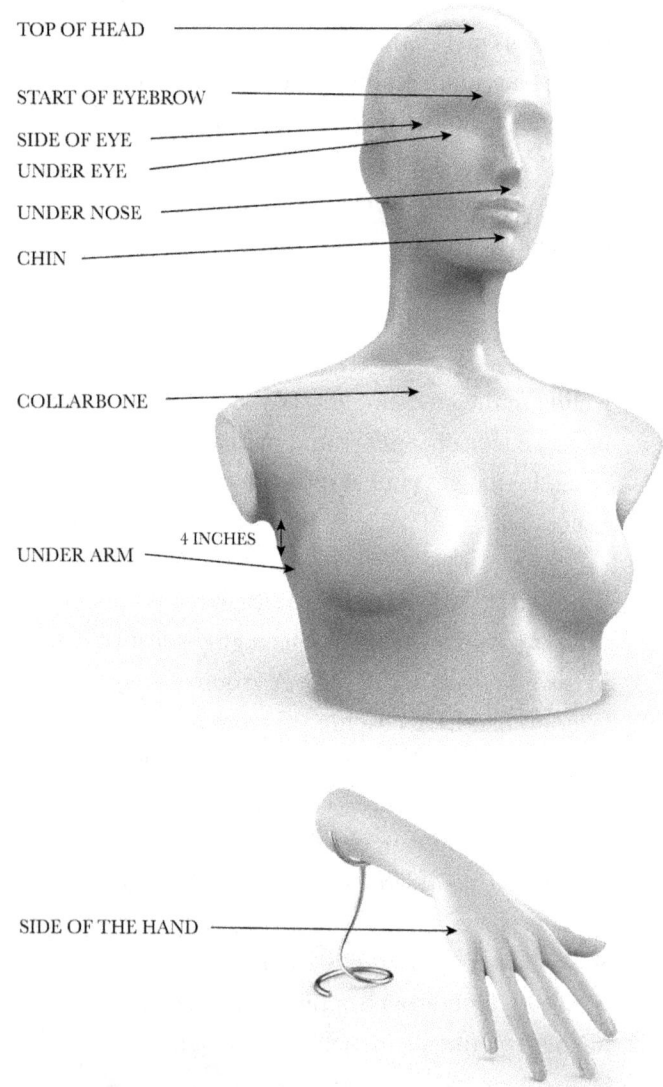

Behavioural Therapy), which are usually therapies that take longer to get results.

How to Tap

You can do a round of tapping in as little as two or three minutes. You do not need any equipment. Find a quiet place where you can sit without interruption.

Step 1: Identify what the issue is and the feeling accompanying it. For example, anxiety over an exam, being overwhelmed regarding revision or even a physical complaint such as a headache.

Try to be specific in how that feels, and where in your body you feel the emotion or 'charge', as we call it.

Step 2: Rate the intensity or severity of the emotion or complaint on a scale of 0–10 (0 = not bothered by it at all, 10 = maximum severity). Go with the first number that comes into your head.

Step 3: Make a statement using this template and inserting the issue you want to work on:

Even though I feel/have............ I choose to accept that part of me.
Example: Even though I feel overwhelmed, I choose to accept this part of me.

Step 4: Say the affirmation aloud while gently rubbing/tapping the side of the hand – the edge of the palm – the part just before the little finger (also known as the *Karate Chop* area).

So, whilst tapping the **Side of the hand**:

- Even though I feel overwhelmed, I choose to accept this part of me.
- Even though I have so much to do and I don't know how I am going to get it done, I choose to accept this part of me.
- Even though I am feeling so stressed right now, I choose to accept this part of me.

Note that we start with the negative first. We do this because we are honouring and acknowledging the feelings, emotions and limiting beliefs that are in existence at that very moment. By doing this we are showing our brains they are not dangerous but they are ready to be cleared.

Now move and tap gently on the different points, ideally six gentle taps on each point before you move on. Really speak how you feel (your 'truth') at this moment in time. This script below is just an example. Use your own words.

Eyebrow: All this anxiety
Side of the eye: All the things I have to do.
Under eye: I'm feeling so scared.
Under nose: Worried I'm not going to get it all done.
Chin: I'm never going to manage it all.
Collarbone: So much to do.
Under arm: I've left it too late to revise.
Top of head: I'm going to fail.
Eyebrow: I am so stressed.
Side of eye: I am so overwhelmed.
Under eye: I don't know what to do with myself.
Under nose: I can't see a way forward.
Chin: I feel so helpless.
Collarbone: All these feelings of overwhelm.
Under arm: Feeling so stressed.
Top of head: So anxious.

Take a break and check in to see if there has been any shift in the number you started off with. If not, continuing tapping with whatever emotions or thoughts come into your head.

Keep going with the tapping until you find that the number you started off with has started to shift downwards – i.e., you are feeling some relief. This might take you a while so keep going.

When you feel you have finished pouring out all the different emotions, thoughts and feelings in your body, you can start to move on to some more positive rounds.

Eyebrow: I now choose to let this overwhelm go.
Side of eye: I have had enough of feeling anxious and stressed.
Under eye: I know what I have to do.
Under nose: I'm going to let this anxiety go.
Chin: I've let it go before; I can do it again.
Collarbone: Being stressed and anxious doesn't actually help me.
Under arm: It just makes me feel worse.
Top of head: I am going to let this stress and overwhelm go.

Eyebrow: Letting it go, starting to release the stress bit by bit.
Side of eye: Releasing all the stress.
Under eye: Releasing the overwhelm.
Under Nose: I am starting to feel better.
Chin: I am starting to feel calm.
Collarbone: I can do this.
Under arm: I can get everything done.
Top of head: I feel calmer.
Eyebrow: It feels better.
Side of eye: I have got this.
Under eye: I can breathe.
Under Nose: I am feeling myself relax a bit more.
Chin: I can do this.
Collarbone: I am doing this.
Underarm: I am okay.

Do you get the idea of this now? Use your own thoughts and emotions as you go through the points. The example above is just an example.

Check in every round and see what your initial number is now. Keep going until you have your number down to a 1 or a 2. This might take a few minutes, or it might take fifteen minutes. There is no set time.

If you do not get down to a 1 or 2 and are tiring, it may be that there are more layers to explore at another time. If new thoughts or emotions come into your head as you are doing this then you can tap on those too as they come up for you.

This exercise might seem a bit unnatural at first, but you'll soon get the hang of it. Keep going with it. If you have the thought 'This isn't going to work for me/Nothing ever works for me', you could start off by doing some tapping to clear this belief and energy away from you as below before you start tapping on any anxiety or worry.

Say out loud to yourself whilst tapping on the side of your hand 'Even though I don't believe this is going to work for me I choose to accept this part of me'.

Or

'Even though nothing ever works for me, I choose to accept this part of me.'

Repeat three times.

Rate the intensity or severity of the emotion on a scale of 0–10. Go with the first number that comes into your head.

Side of hand: Even though I get *angry/cross/frustrated/sad* that nothing works for me, I choose to accept this part of me *(choose the emotions and feelings that resonate with you).*
Side of hand: Even though I sometimes start something but do not complete it, I choose to accept this part of me.
Side of hand: Even though I am anxious because nothing works for me, I choose to relax now.
Eyebrow: Nothing ever works.
Side of eye: I have tried so many different things.
Under eye: And none have ever worked for me.
Under nose: Nothing ever works.
Chin: So why should this?
Collarbone: Why should this be any different?
Under arm: It might work for others but not for me.
Top of head: I'm so frustrated/angry/cross/sad.

Check in and see what score you are on now. If the score hasn't shifted down, do a few more rounds of whatever is coming up for you. Again, the above is only an example; use words and feelings that are bothering you.

When you feel some relief and a shift you can go towards a positive round, but remember not to force this; it has to feel natural to you so take your time with this and if you get a feeling of 'I don't believe this' or 'it isn't true' you may need to do some more rounds tapping on these thoughts before moving on as below.

Eyebrow: I am choosing to open myself up to the possibility that this may work.
Side of eye: I am allowing myself to believe that there may be something in this that can help me.
Under eye: I can feel my body start to relax as I say this.
Under nose: Things have worked for me before.
Chin: I have made positive changes in the past.
Collarbone: I can change.

Under arm: I can choose to make changes.
Top of head: I can release that frustration/anger.
Eyebrow: I feel myself letting go of the tension.
Under eye: Letting go of the belief this can't work for me.
Under nose: Letting it all go.
Chin: I am starting to allow the belief that this can work for me.
Collarbone: I can feel myself relaxing and shifting.
Under arm: Allowing myself to believe it can help me.
Top of head: I am choosing my ability to change.

Note how you are now feeling. Repeat this exercise as often as you need.

How can this help during exams? It can release anxious feelings and emotions and bring you back to a sense of calm and control.

Journalling & Automatic or Free Writing

The aim of journalling is to express and capture your thoughts and feelings on paper. You might want to think of it as a 'brain dump'. The act of transferring thoughts onto paper can make it easier to let go of anxious thoughts. It can stop you ruminating, can put things in perspective and help organise your thinking.

You can allocate a journal or notepad to do this, and you can even doodle, colour or draw if you are not so keen on using the written word. Write down anything that comes to mind. If you are stuck it can be helpful to put down how your day is going, what you are thinking and how you are feeling. Do not stress about it being perfect or over the spelling or grammar; just let the words flow. Continue until you come to a natural end.

You can go back to review what you have written and challenge some of your thoughts with questions such as:

- Is this true? Do I really believe this?
- Could I think of this differently? From a different perspective?
- Could there be something positive from this? If so, what might it be?
- Think about your strengths and how you handled difficult situations before. What can you draw on from those experiences now?
- What could you change or do differently?
- What resources could you draw upon?
- What are you learning from this?

If you find this practice helpful you might like to make this part of your daily routine before your day starts (this has been called 'Morning Pages' for that reason). It can be great for mental clarity and setting your intention for the day – this is my favourite time of day to write – but you can do it in the evening, or otherwise just when you are drawn to it.

Automatic Writing

Automatic writing is a slightly different version of journalling. It usually follows a short meditative practice. The aim here is to go into a deep state of relaxation before you start writing. This can be useful for focusing on a specific question or issue that is bothering you and that you would like to know the answer to. It allows you to tap into your inner wisdom, intuition and the creativity of your subconscious mind. You then write down the responses as they come to you, so you can gain guidance on the question or problem you are grappling with.

Steps for Automatic Writing

1. Set aside half an hour or so. You might want to set a timer if you only have a certain amount of time to do this (you may get so caught up in the flow here that you do not realise the time has gone by, so an alarm can help here).

2. Find a quiet space where you are not going to be interrupted. Sit down comfortably. You might like to have essential oils around you and/or some candles and some light mellow music in the background. Or you may prefer silence. Have your journal (online or paper) ready, with a new page open, ready to go.

3. Focus your attention on a question or an area that has been troubling you or that you want the answer to. It is helpful as well to set an intention of what part of yourself that you would like to tap into – for example, your subconscious mind or your heart or inner guidance (sometimes called the Higher Self), whichever you resonate most with.

The question might be something general such as 'What do I need to know today? What are my next steps with regard to x, y, z?' (Avoid asking yes or no questions.)

Or, you might want to know the answer to something specific such as 'Dear Higher Self, why do I get so anxious? What do I need to know about my anxiety? What is going to help me?'

Choose one question for now. You can always come back and ask another question next time. Keep it simple!

4. Now relax your body and mind. You can do this by taking three deep breaths in through the nose and then exhale through the mouth.

As you are breathing in, imagine, sense or feel you are breathing in peace and calmness. As you exhale set the intention to breathe out and release any stress, anxiety or tension. Breathe in this way for a few cycles until you feel completely relaxed. Then just go back to your regular breathing pattern.

5. Now feel yourself becoming very present in the moment, becoming aware of the weight of your body against the chair or bed supporting you and any sounds in the background.

6. Set the intention to let go of any worries from your day. Take another deep breath in and let it go out of the mouth.

7. Start writing immediately and just allow the words and answers to flow. Write down everything that comes to you. Subconscious inspirations are often subtle so do not question or judge what you are writing, just go with it, even if it doesn't make total sense to you.

The process should just feel light and easy, flowing, as if the pen is just moving across the page, almost as if you are not aware of writing.

Tools to Get Us Back into Safe and Social

Continue writing until you naturally come to an end. Do not stop part way and go back and look at what you have written.

8. When you feel nothing more is coming to you, review what you have written. You might like to highlight anything that stands out for you, any word, sentence or any clear guidance.

Words from your heart, intuition and Higher Self will *always* feel kind, loving and positive.

If you are not sure about anything it might become clear to you later (our brains can take time to process information), you can use your next automatic writing session to seek further clarity and guidance.

The more you practice automatic writing or journalling the easier it becomes, and the more you will trust the process and what comes from it. It is about becoming more aware of oneself and building up a trusted friendship and relationship.

'When my life is going well, I live it, when it isn't I write it.'

– G Vilas, tennis pro

I believe you can also write when things are going well. You can magnify that energy and gain new insights and opportunities.

How can this help with exams? Writing during stressful times can be useful to express and release negative emotions, thoughts and anxiety. It can help you connect with yourself, explore your emotions and patterns and clarify your thinking. Just putting things down on paper can bring a different perspective and help you to feel calmer.

Intuitive Painting/Drawing

Just as automatic writing is meditation with words, intuitive painting or drawing could be described as 'meditating with a brush or pencil in your hand'. It is a heartfelt and guided self-exploration through art/paint/sculpture/drawing, deepening the connection with oneself.

There is no set formula as to how to begin.

You might want to follow steps 1 to 6 above in *Automatic Writing*, and then just start to paint or draw shapes, symbols, and add colour — whatever comes to you.

How can this help with exams? It can allow you to express anxiety and painful emotions and thoughts that you are not able to put into words. It can also give you space from unwanted feelings and allow you to focus on something that you can control. It also brings you into the present moment.

Anxiety-Busting Diet

Diet can really make a difference to our mood and energy. Think of a car that has dirty or substandard petrol or fuel put into it. The engine splutters and can finally grind to a halt. The same for our bodies. As a certified health coach and having studied nutrition I know the importance diet can make and the effect it has on mental, emotional and physical wellbeing.

In the run up to exams, think about what you eat and try to include lots of anti-anxiety foods. These are some of my top choices:

- Salad (celery, cucumber. lettuce).
- Vegetables (broccoli, carrots, kale, spinach, Swiss Chard).
- Healthy fats such as avocados, olive oil, butter, coconut oil.
- Lean protein (grass-fed beef, poultry, wild-caught fish, organic or free-range eggs, if budget allows, tofu).
- Nuts (almonds, Brazil nuts, pecans, cashews, walnuts) and seeds (pumpkin, sunflower, flax, chia) – These are a great source of protein, especially for vegans and vegetarians.
- Lentils.
- Fermented foods, such as kimchi, sauerkraut and kefir, are great for gut health.
- Whole grains.
- Berries (these are the lowest sugar fruit options).
- And for that occasional treat, dark chocolate. Choose one with the highest cacao content you can tolerate and minimal sugar content.

Exam Day Meals

Research has shown that those who eat breakfast perform better. Even if you do not usually eat breakfast, try to east something on exam day, even if it is just a piece of fruit. It gives you energy. Ideally for breakfast you want some slow-release carbohydrates like wholegrain oats or wholegrain bread and some protein such as eggs to keep you full longer. If you can add in some omega-3 fatty acids, such as avocado, salmon or other fatty fish, even better, as our brain is around 60% fat, and this will give it a boost.

Some breakfast ideas include the following:

- Scrambled or poached egg on wholegrain toast with smoked salmon, spinach and avocado on the side.
- Omelette with ham or cheese, tomato and mushrooms.
- Wholegrain oats with seeds, nuts and berries (this can be nice if you do overnight oats and soak in milk (non-dairy milk such as coconut or almond if you are intolerant to dairy). Frozen berries can be used too and are often higher in nutritional content than those on the fresh shelves in supermarkets that may have been in transit for days. Freezing shortly after picking allows them

to retain their antioxidant content better. Add dried fruit or some organic honey if you need it to be a little sweeter.
- Sugar-free muesli or granola topped with yoghurt or milk of your choice and berries.
- Natural yoghurt with banana or sliced apple, berries, grapes, seeds and nuts.
- A smoothie with banana or avocado as the base, adding in different fruits and vegetables.

If you have an exam in the afternoon, choose what you are going to eat for lunch with care too. Too heavy a meal will make you feel laden down and sleepy. We don't want that, do we?

My favourite meal during my A Levels (many years ago now, but I still remember it vividly as it really worked for me) was an open-faced salad sandwich with wholegrain bread. I'd have different salad and protein toppings (chicken, ham, tuna, salmon, smoked mackerel, sardines, smoked salmon or a boiled egg), followed by some fruit. I felt full but light after and it became my exam staple as I knew I could trust it as a nutritious meal that wasn't going to upset my stomach and digestion.

Foods to avoid:
- Fried food.
- Trans fats (vegetable oil, canola, sunflower oil).
- Gluten, if you feel you might be sensitive to it.
- Cakes, pastries.
- Sugar.
- Processed food.
- Fizzy and soda drinks.
- Artificial sweeteners.
- Avoid turkey on the day of an exam as it contains L-tryptophan that may make you feel sleepy!

A Note on Sugar

Sugar is a big one. Yes, it is found naturally in fruits, which are extremely good for us, but here I am really talking about high fructose content sugar, which seems to be hidden in almost everything we eat today.

If you are craving sugar, look behind it to see what it is you are actually looking for. It is more than likely to be an emotional need rather than a physical one. For me, sugar metaphorically represents the sweetness of life, so how can you give that sweetness to yourself, without indulging in that treat? It might be playing some music or giving the dog or cat, if you have one, some attention.

Sugar is fine for an occasional treat, but it could be making your anxiety worse if you consume a lot of sugary food. If you do need something sweet, I prefer to add some honey or a drop of maple syrup to a dish. Have a handful of blueberries – even frozen ones in the summer – as a sweet treat. They're great brain food too.

Caffeine

Caffeine, the chemical found in tea, coffee, chocolate and energy drinks, is a stimulant, which kicks our nervous system into action, keeping us awake, alert and warding off tiredness. Although, on the one hand, this might be a benefit for revision, you may be one of the many people who are sensitive to caffeine, experiencing nervousness, jittery feelings and a racing heart. It can put you in that fight or flight state and cause or worsen anxiety. So just a note of caution. It can help with alertness, but it will depend on how sensitive you are to it.

Caffeine may also impair sleep, which is very important during exam time. We know the temptation can be to condense the hours we sleep to get more revision time in. To avoid any negative impact on sleep, limit your caffeine intake, especially after midafternoon, and replace it with herbal tea, green tea or water. We will talk more about sleep a bit further on.

Drink Water

Our bodies, depending on our gender, weight, and height, are more than fifty percent water. The bottom line is that we all need to be hydrated for our bodies to operate to the optimum. If we do not drink enough water, it can lead to low concentration and, sometimes, we might experience a slight headache. So, staying hydrated before and during exams is especially key for good brain function.

You can tell if you are hydrated by looking at your pee. You ideally want it to be light in colour (not dark). Note that some medications and supplements, like vitamins C and B, can make your urine a brighter colour. That is perfectly natural.

If you are not that keen on just plain water, then you might like to add some fruits such as berries or apples, or cucumber or celery. Some tea brands make fruit infusions. I make a big jug up and have it cold with ice in the summer. I sip it during the day, knowing that I am getting sufficient liquid and without having to get repeat refills.

Avoid:
- Energy drinks and fizzy drinks, soda and fruit juices. Often high in sugar or sweeteners, they can promote blood and energy spikes and heighten anxiety.
- Caffeine (if it makes you jittery) – see the section on caffeine above for more information.

Vitamin, Mineral and Herbal Supplements

Although I like to use food as my main source of nutrients and minerals, there are times when we don't get all that we need from our food. Some anxiety symptoms may be eased through supplementation. Vitamins B and D, omega-3 fatty acids and magnesium can be key in helping balance our moods. Herbs can help too. If you want to explore further, speak to your parent or carer and consult a medical professional on what might be at play for you and for their targeted recommendations. Supplements can have side effects and can interact with other medications you might be taking so **you should only take them under the advice and guidance of a medical professional.**

Traditional Medications for Anxiety

Medication can have its place and sometimes it is necessary, especially as a short-term solution, to get young people through a particularly bad period of depression and anxiety. However, it can just mask the symptoms, the root cause of which might be trauma based, caused by gut imbalance, or neurotransmitter or hormone imbalance (more than likely a combination of some of these). If you suspect that any of these may be at the root of your anxiety, please consult your doctor.

I understand it is not a decision anyone takes lightly, so if you do take prescription medication, do so under the guidance of a medical practitioner/GP who can support and review your ongoing needs with you.

Exercise

Physical exercise releases powerful endorphins, which are mood lifting and have been proven to help reduce anxiety and panic attacks.

Ideally, you should exercise regularly – twenty to thirty minutes, five times a week – and try to move your body every day. Whatever you choose – gentle stretching, yoga, Pilates, Tai Chi, running, fitness classes, dancing, weight training, tennis, group sports like football, rugby, netball, hockey, swimming, rowing, boxing, cross fit, HIT – any form of exercise is good for you.

Exercise can be a great distraction, diverting your attention from what is worrying you. It is also incredibly useful to re-energise in between revision periods and after exams. It really gets the blood and those feel-good endorphins flowing.

Note, however, that exercise, if excessive, can add stress to an already depleted body, so just be aware of this. Moderation is recommended if you are low in energy or suffer from fatigue.

Walking in Nature

This is a go-to favourite for me. Being out in nature, whether that is in a forest, mountains or at the beach, is a wonderful way to instantly de-stress. Immersing yourself in your surroundings and using all your senses – sight, smell, hearing, etc. – can be extremely calming. Research shows that some tree compounds can decrease stress hormone levels. And birdsong can help mental health. Some hospitals play recorded birdsong to children before their operations as they have found that it helps calm nerves. You might want to listen to recorded birdsong – find some online – before an exam.

Mindful Walking Meditation

Unable to sit and meditate but still want the well-documented benefits? Did you know you can turn a walk into a mindful meditation? Yes, you heard me – you don't need to sit in silence to meditate (which I know puts so many people off). Just begin by taking in your surroundings and being fully present as you walk. When we are fully present and focused just on that moment, our minds cannot ruminate about the past or wander into worry about the future.

Here is a mini routine you can follow or adapt as you see fit.

1. Start by focussing on how it feels as your feet hit the ground. What part of your foot lands first and how do your toes, soles and heels feel? How do your feet feel in the shoes you are wearing? What sounds are your shoes or boots making on the ground? How does the ground feel beneath your feet? Solid? Soft?

How does the impact of walking go up through your ankles, calves and your thighs? Do the muscles feel tight or relaxed? How about your hips? How are they moving and feeling? Note how they are connected to your pelvis and your abdomen.

2. Next, notice what your arms are doing. Are they naturally swinging as you are walking?

How are you holding your hands? How are they feeling? Warm? Cool?

What about your head and neck? Your back and spine, stomach and chest? Is there tightness there? If so, just notice it and maybe breathe into that area, if it feels okay to do so, with more conscious deeper breathing.

3. Then start to really notice your surroundings: the assorted colours of the trees and flowers, how the trees move in the breeze. Go and touch some of the leaves of the trees and plants. Notice the shade or colour tone and feel their texture.

What colour is the sky? How does it look? Bright, cloudy, grey, stormy?

What can you smell? What does the temperature feel like on any exposed skin? Your face? Your hands?

What sounds are you hearing? What is grabbing your attention most? Zoom in on what else can you hear behind the most obvious things in the background noises.

What is the temperature like? How does the outside air feel as you breathe it in? Is it cool? Warm? How does it feel as it enters your lungs? How is your body taking in the breath? Are you breathing deeply? Easily? And if you change pace, just notice with interest how your breath changes.

4. Tap into how you are feeling. Can you name the emotion you are feeling? Where are you feeling it in the body? How do the feelings shift?

Focusing on identifying the feelings in our bodies helps with anxiety. Many of us try to go into our minds and try to outthink anxiety. Concentrating on the body can help us get out of our heads for a while.

Most importantly, just relax and enjoy the moment and breathe! Take a deep breath in through your nose and inhale the peace and calmness. As you exhale, let go of any tension or anything that is now ready to be released. Do this for another couple of deep breaths. Enjoy all the elements of your walk.

You might want to add some gratitude for the surroundings and for your body, your legs for supporting you, your feet for grounding you, your eyes for all you can see, your ears for all you can hear, etc. You get the idea?

Grounding

Grounding (sometimes called earthing) is all about connecting to the frequency and natural electromagnetics of the earth and nature. It is believed that the electrical charges of the earth can benefit our health. Research is limited, but the studies that have been done report that people who practice grounding feel better, more connected to themselves, and that it can help mood.

The best way to ground is to walk outside barefoot, your feet touching the grass, soil or sand. Lay your palms on the earth too. You can even lie on the ground, increasing the skin to surface contact you have with the earth. This is one of the reasons gardening can be therapeutic. Getting your hands into the soil is a great way to connect with the earth.

How can this help during exams? It can be great to do before an exam to just re-balance yourself. And, if you tend to dissociate (feeling floaty, spacy, as if you are outside of your body), grounding can immediately bring you back into feeling more connected to yourself and the world.

Sleep

Getting a good night's sleep is non-negotiable. However, when we are anxious it can be hard to fall asleep or stay asleep. We can wake in the early hours, full of worry, unable to fall back to sleep again. And then we worry about not being able to sleep. It can be a vicious cycle. We all know how groggy we can feel after a disturbed night, both physically and mentally.

Think of sleep increasing brainpower just as weightlifting or training builds our muscles.

Sleep is one of those things that, during exams, can really suffer with students studying and revising into the early hours. If you are a night owl you might be able to do this, but if you are a morning person you are better off getting a good night's sleep and getting up early in the morning, when you are fresh, to continue your studies.

The night before an exam I recommend you try not to study too late. There's evidence that students who sleep for seven hours a night do, on average, 10% better than those who get less sleep.

If you find you are struggling to sleep, I have found reverse psychology to be helpful, so try to keep yourself awake. That actually makes it easier to fall asleep. Rather than tossing and turning you might want to take the pressure off and get up and maybe make a warm drink or read (not your revision notes but some light fiction perhaps) until you feel sleepy. I will also listen to a calming meditation or sleep meditation. If I can't get off to sleep, or if I wake in the night, I find that helpful. We are all different though, so find what works for you.

To set yourself up for a good night's sleep:
- Do not have a heavy evening meal and try to finish eating at least two to three hours

before you go to bed to allow for your meal to be digested. Your body then does not have to use up vital energy in digesting the food whilst you sleep.
- If you need a snack before bed, a banana or a handful of almonds or nuts is a good option.
- Do not drink too much liquid before bed, and no caffeine. If budget allows there are some nighttime herbal tea infusions that are great. Otherwise check out my calming Golden Tea recipe in *Resources* at the back of this book.
- A warm bath or shower can help relax you. Add in a drop of a relaxing essential oil or some Epsom salts.
- Turn off electronics and, if possible, leave your phone outside the bedroom. If you need an alarm, use a standalone alarm clock so you do not need your phone.
- Read or listen to music to relax before you switch off for the night.

Your bedroom ideally should be:
- At a temperature between 60 and 70 degrees F.
- Clutter-free (clear room, clear mind).
- Decorated in relaxing colours.

- Dark (I recommend blackout blinds/curtains) – if you do need a light at night try to make it a dimmed night light (bright light can interfere with melatonin production, waking us up, and we can find it hard to get back to sleep).

Last thing before you go to sleep, I recommend you spend a few minutes mentally reviewing your day, focusing on all the positives and highlights. This ends the day on a positive tone and can set the mood nicely for waking up the next day with an optimistic outlook.

Essential Oils/Aromatherapy

Essential oils are natural liquid extracts from the flowers, leaves, stems, roots and bark of plants. Some, such as lavender and chamomile, are believed to be helpful for calming anxiety and promoting relaxation and sleep. Others, such as lemon and peppermint, are thought to aid mental focus and concentration. My favourite way of experiencing their benefits is through using a diffuser. Before using, however, please consult your local health shop and/or a trained aromatherapist as they will be able to advise you on usage, brands and suitable choices for you. Never ingest essential oils.

Crystals for Anxiety and Stress Relief

Despite limited scientific evidence, crystals have been used down the centuries for their professed healing properties for the body, mind and soul. It is believed that their energy vibrates at a higher frequency than we humans, positively influencing our energy and mood.

Many of my younger clients believe that crystals have helped them with anxiety. Remember that your beliefs become your reality and, if you believe they help you, then that will be your experience.

Below are some of the most common crystals and their properties.

Smokey Quartz – for feeling grounded, safe and secure, especially during periods of great stress.

Rose Quartz – for unconditional love, self-compassion and forgiveness of self and others.

Black Tourmaline – for grounding during periods of worry or strain and absorption of negative energy.

Citrine – for self-esteem and reduction of panic attacks.

Amethyst – to calm the nerves and balance emotions, bringing a sense of peace.

Black obsidian – for panic attacks and to help counteract negative energy from electromagnetic frequencies (EMFs).

Shungite – for cleansing of mind and body and shielding against EMFs – great for protection when you're on your phone or other electrical devices.

Aquamarine – to calm and reduces stress.

Blue Lace Agate – for calming nerves and reducing stress.

Carnelian – to let go of negative thoughts.

Jade – to balance emotions and promote inner tranquillity.

Usually, you will be drawn to a particular crystal. It is as though it chooses you. So, if you are looking at a bowl of crystals, just see which one catches your eye. Pick it up and see how it feels to you.

How to use crystals

Crystals need to be cleansed regularly to remove stagnant energy. You can submerge them in salt water or leave them outside in the moonlight. Some, but not all, can be left out in direct sunlight – check before you do this. There are great books and sites on the internet that will tell you how to do this.

You can then 'programme' your crystal to enhance its effectiveness. Hold it in your hand and focus your mind on the way you'd like it to help you. For example, you can set the intention for the crystal to keep you feeling safe and calm, help you with concentration as you revise, keep you clear of other people's negativity and tension, etc.

You can wear crystals as jewellery, keep them in a pocket or put them on your desk when studying or revising. You can also have them around you to help with meditation. Or hold them in your palm as *worry stones* to provide comfort.

Calming Basket

You might like to think about pulling together a Calming Basket or box of things you can turn to when you need a little bit of reassurance and comfort. This might contain a list of your affirmations, essential oils for calming, or it might be where you keep your journal or a notepad to jot down any worries you have. There might be some comforting words or a poem, a colouring book or your crystals, a stress ball or worry beads, or a cuddly toy from childhood. You can put anything in here that you can call upon when you need a little bit of help to calm down.

Seeking Professional Help

Please know that there are highly trained professionals out there to help you cope with your anxiety, if it gets to a level where you feel that you could do with outside assistance. So, please reach out for help if you need it. A couple of modalities you might like to explore are described below.

Clinical hypnotherapy

Clinical hypnotherapy can really help, especially to get to the root cause of what might be causing your anxiety or panic attacks. Often the cause is a subconscious incident or incidents in our past. Working with a qualified hypnotherapist, as we have said, can uncover limiting beliefs, thoughts and can reprogramme your brain to adopt new ways of thinking and patterns of behaviour. There are no side effects.

Cognitive Behavioural therapy (CBT)

In this book we have looked at reframing thoughts and the way you perceive events and how your body reacts to them. Working with a CBT therapist you'd work more deeply to identify your own personal patterns with a view to changing how you think and react to situations. So, for example, instead of panicking about an exam, you reframe it as a chance to show how much you have learned.

The most important thing for me as a therapist and as someone who combines many of the above modalities and tools we have looked at is that you work with someone you have rapport with and trust and who comes from an approved body. This is key. Do think about whether you prefer to see someone in person, face to face, or are happy to work online. I work internationally and conduct a lot of my sessions online, and the results are just as effective as in person. It is a matter of personal choice. There may be some free resources too that you can access via your doctor.

Please do not feel that asking for help is an admission of weakness. We are all on this earth to help one another and there is no shame in asking for help. In fact, it is a sign of strength.

Self-harm and Suicidal Thoughts

With regards to self-harm and suicide, we need to get this conversation out there. We need to address this as a society. All of us, at some time or other in our lives, are likely to go through a period when we feel overwhelmed, we can't see a way forward and we want to escape.

I felt it important to include a section here to help you if you are feeling overwhelmed, or if you suspect that a loved one or friend is self-harming or having suicidal thoughts.

First of all, please know that you are not alone in this. Your feelings are your feelings. We have talked in this book about how important it is to acknowledge our darker thoughts and emotions. There is no shame in having these feelings or admitting you have them. It is a sign of being human and it takes courage and strength to admit you need help or assistance.

Secondly, there are people out there who can offer that help and assistance. I've included information about those organisations below. Many of them operate 24/7. Please, please, please talk to someone you trust about how you are feeling. Because it does not have to be this way. There is no shame in seeking help. If you're thinking about suicide, or actively planning how to die by suicide, talking to a loved one or therapist about such thoughts is the first step to overcoming them, strengthening mental well-being and moving toward recovery. What have you got to lose?

Self-harm

Self-harm can be a way of coping with difficult feelings – to feel physical pain, to distract from emotional pain, to stop feeling 'numb' and to release tension. Remember we talked about how we can dissociate in Part

One, as it can be too difficult to be in our body. Self-harm is a coping mechanism and a habit that is hard to stop. Please do seek advice from an adult if you suspect someone you know is self-harming.

Ways that young people self-harm include:
- Cutting themselves.
- Scratching skin with fingernails.
- Burning skin.
- Biting skin.
- Hitting themselves or banging their head or another part of their body on a wall.
- Pulling hair out from their head, eyebrows or eyelashes.
- Inserting objects into their body.

Signs to look out for include:
- Unexplained cuts, burns, bite marks, bruises or bald patches.
- Keeping themselves covered – for example, wearing long sleeves or trousers even during hot weather, not wanting to change clothes around others or avoiding activities like swimming.
- An excessive amount of tissues in waste bins.

- Seeming low or depressed – for example, withdrawing from friends and family.
- Blaming themselves for problems or expressing feelings of failure, uselessness or hopelessness.
- Outbursts of anger or argumentativeness.

While self-harm often may provide relief in the moment, this relief is temporary. As feelings build up again, so does the desire to self-harm, and it can become a pattern that is hard to escape from. This can lead to feelings of shame, guilt, confusion and fear, adding to the stress load of what you are already going through. Please note that the STOP process we talked about earlier may be helpful here. I recommend you do consult a professional therapist, who will be able to help.

Suicidal thoughts

I am going to share something very personal to me. This last year, I lost an extremely good friend and mentor. He took his own life. He seemingly had the world at his feet. His suicide came as a complete shock to all of us, even those closest to him. None of us had any idea of the pain he was in. His death and the circumstances of it are devastating and I am writing this, with heartfelt sincerity, to highlight to those who are in such deep need that there is a way forward. My friend kept it so hidden that no one had any inkling. He did not give us the chance to help support him. We need to talk about our feelings and about self-harm and suicide. It is time to speak out about it and to help break down the stigma surrounding it and mental health.

What to do if you suspect someone is struggling

Many of us, understandably, are not sure what to do in this situation if we do suspect someone we love is struggling and self-harming or contemplating suicide.

There may be signs, which may include:
- Talks about feeling hopeless, worthless, trapped or talking about not having a reason to keep living or says things such as 'I wish I'd never been born'.
- Searches for means to self-harm, such as how to access medications.
- Sleeps too little or too much.
- Eats too little or too much.

- Shows signs of despair or has significant mood swings.
- Acts agitated, anxious or aggressive.
- Avoids other people, including loved ones; spends more time than usual alone.
- Behaves recklessly.
- Drinks alcohol or uses drugs excessively.
- Has experienced a severe life stressor recently, such as the death of a spouse, the loss of a job or a traumatic event.
- Has attempted suicide or demonstrated suicidal behaviour in the past.

However, none of these might be present, so, if you have a sense or a feeling that something is a bit 'off', ask the individual outright if they are having suicidal thoughts. Despite widespread fears about asking directly if someone is contemplating suicide, it will not put the idea in their head if it was not there to begin with. Most people are grateful and relieved that someone has raised the topic with them. And even if they are indignant, you can trust that you have done the right thing and been a good friend by starting a conversation that needed to be had.

If the person does admit that they are feeling suicidal, get them help as soon as possible. Do not leave them alone for a moment. If you can't be with them yourself, get someone else to go and be with them, or keep talking to them on the phone if you are not physically present. Take them to the emergency department of your local hospital as soon as you can.

Useful UK Contact Numbers

Unless it says otherwise, they're open 24 hours a day, every day. You can also call these helplines for advice for yourself or if you're worried about someone else.

Information

Samaritans – for everyone
https://www.samaritans.org/
Call 116 123
Email jo@samaritans.org

Campaign Against Living Miserably (CALM)
https://www.thecalmzone.net/
Call 0800 58 58 58 – 5pm to midnight every day
Visit https://www.thecalmzone.net/help/webchat/ for the webchat page
https://www.thecalmzone.net/get-support

Papyrus – prevention of young suicide
HOPELINE247
https://www.papyrus-uk.org/useful-health-apps/
HOPELINE247
Call 0800 068 41 41
Text 07860 039967
Email pat@papyrus-uk.org

Childline – for children and young people under 19
Call 0800 1111 – the number will not show up on your phone bill
https://www.childline.org.uk/

SOS Silence of Suicide – for everyone
https://sossilenceofsuicide.org/
Call 0300 1020 505 – 4pm to midnight every day
Email support@sossilenceofsuicide.org

Message a text line

If you do not want to talk to someone over the phone, these text lines are open 24 hours a day, every day:

Shout Crisis Text Line – for everyone
Text SHOUT to 85258
https://giveusashout.org/

YoungMinds Crisis Messenger – for people under 19
Text YM to 85258
https://www.youngminds.org.uk/young-person/shout-85258/

Self Injury Support webchat (for women/girls) – open Tuesday, Wednesday and Thursday from 7 pm to 9:30 pm
https://www.selfinjurysupport.org.uk/Pages/FAQs/Category/webchat-support

CALM webchat (for men/boys) – open from 5 pm to midnight every day
https://www.thecalmzone.net/get-support

Mind – How to help someone with suicidal feelings

https://www.mind.org.uk/information-support/helping-someone-else/supporting-someone-who-feels-suicidal/how-to-help/

Summary of Part Two

In Part Two we have explored practical tools and techniques to mitigate and, hopefully, in many cases eradicate that deep anxiety and nervousness about revision and exams. These are tried and trusted techniques that I have found work with my clients, with the aim to get you back into that *safe and social* state, and feeling of safety, that we talked about in Part One.

We explored revision tips and diet, and the importance of diet for good brain function, concentration and focus.

Summary of Part Two

We looked at our negative thinking patterns and tendencies and looked at exercises to help reframe these. We introduced the STOP technique. We also explored the notion that emotions are *energy in motion* and that different emotions vibrate at different frequencies, with shame at the lower end and joy and love at the high end. We explored that emotions come and go every ninety seconds or so and that 'if we can see it we can shift it'.

We have explored mindfulness, breathwork and meditation, hypnosis and affirmations. We also looked at using crystals.

We have talked about the importance of reaching out for help if you need it, that it is not a sign of weakness but one of strength and courage. We noted some useful therapies to look at and, most importantly, what to do if you or someone you know is contemplating suicide.

Bringing my top recommendations together in one place:

Easing Exam Nerves Daily Protocol

- Upon waking, set the tone and intention for the day: 'Today is going to be a good day' and affirmations and positive 'What ifs…'
- Mindful breathing practice in moments of anxiety/worry/panic.
- Balanced diet.
- Watch your thoughts and language and reframe negative ones.
- Meditation, gratitude, journalling – a practice that allows you to connect with yourself.
- Mild to moderate exercise (too much can add to stress load).
- Do something that brings you fun and joy or something you love to do.
- Address sleep issues.
- At bedtime – affirmations and pick out the positive things that happened that day.

I hope that, within this book, you have found some relief. I also hope that you feel comforted in the knowledge that you are not alone.

Remember that weather comes and goes, but the sunshine is always there, even if we cannot see it at the time.

Conclusion and Moving Forwards

So, we have come to the end of our journey together. I hope for you this is a beginning of a new way to look at things and that some of the theories and tools and techniques have helped you – not only to know yourself better but to learn what particularly works for you and your anxiety. And, most importantly, to realise that there is a way forward.

I have so loved sharing with you all the knowledge I have accumulated. I would love to know what has worked for you, if there is anything I have missed. Please reach out if you have your own tips that we can perhaps share with others.

In the meantime, I wish you heartfelt success with your exams. Remember 'this time too shall pass'.

With heartfelt thanks and all the best in your exams going forwards. You've got this! And please do gift or pass on this book to anyone who you feel may need it.

Thank you! Thank you! Thank you!

Resources

Anti-Exam-Anxiety Smoothie

This mood stabilizing healthy chocolate-blueberry smoothie is a delicious, guilt-free treat that is perfect for breakfast, dessert or a snack. It's easy enough to whip up with basic ingredients from your kitchen, and you can always add different berries, protein powder or more greens and, of course, leave out the nuts if you are allergic!

Ingredients

- 1 1/2 cups coconut water or milk of your choice
- 1 Tbsp coconut oil (optional – a good source of Omega-3 fatty acids)
- 1/2 cup frozen blueberries (known as brain berries in some quarters)
- 1/4 avocado or small banana
- 2 Tbsp cocoa powder or 1 oz dark chocolate

Optional

- 1/4 cup Greek yoghurt
- 2 handfuls spinach or greens powder (optional)
- 1 Tbsp protein powder, vanilla or chocolate flavour – avoid whey protein powder if you are dairy intolerant)

Pinch of cinnamon
Pinch of ginger
Pinch of turmeric

Instructions
1. Combine all ingredients in blender at high speed until smooth (usually about 45 to 60 seconds).

2. Add more liquid until you have the consistency you like.

Notes from Alison
1. Make extra smoothie in a glass container like an old spaghetti jar or Mason jar to enjoy for an afternoon snack, dinner or breakfast the next morning. Smoothies are not as nutritious on day two, but still healthy and good for 24 hours. Shake in jar before serving. Bottom line, do what works for you!

2. Freeze some to enjoy at a later date or when you are pushed for time.

Comforting Bedtime Golden Tea/Latte

This is drunk a lot in Asia and is known as 'liquid gold'. I love a cup of this as part of my wind-down bed routine too – so nourishing and silky smooth, and so good for you.

Ingredients

- 1 cup of milk of your choice (I like almond or coconut milk)
- 1 tsp turmeric
- 1 tsp ground ginger
- 1/2 tsp black pepper (this helps the absorption of the turmeric)
- 1/2 tsp cinnamon (optional)

Instructions

Warm all the ingredients through in a saucepan for a few minutes and serve when hot (just before it boils).

Notes from Alison

1. I find this sweet enough as it is but add some honey (make sure it is raw) to sweeten to taste, as necessary.

2. Turmeric is one of the most powerful and most studied herbs of all time. There are over 6,000 research articles on turmeric for its benefits, due to its active compound, curcumin.

3. If you do not have access to all of these ingredients, a cup of warm milk of your choice can be very comforting by itself.

Extra Reading Materials, References and Resources

Preface

Pressure of exams causing worrying levels of anxiety in students, Rebecca Coxon, mentalhealthy.co.uk
https://www.mentalhealthy.co.uk/news/321-pressure-of-exams-causing-worrying-levels-of-anxiety-in-students.html

Children and stress, what's worrying them most, childrenscommissioner.gov.uk
https://www.childrenscommissioner.gov.uk/blog/children-and-stress-whats-worrying-them-most/

Part One
You are not alone/Anxiety and Academic Performance

Anxiety's Hidden Cost In Academic Performance, anxietyreliefsolutions.com
https://anxietyreliefsolutions.com/anxietys-hidden-cost-in-academic-performance/

Disassociation

What is dissociation? MIND mental health website
https://www.mind.org.uk/information-support/types-of-mental-health-problems/dissociation-and-dissociative-disorders/about-dissociation/

Safe and Social States

Polyvagal Theory: How Our Vagus Nerve Controls Responses to our Environment, Jodi Clarke, MA, LPC/MHSP, verywellmind.com
https://www.verywellmind.com/polyvagal-theory-4588049

What is The Polyvagal Theory? Stephen W. Porges, PhD, Polyvagal Theory, stephenporges.com
https://www.polyvagalinstitute.org/whatispolyvagaltheory

Extra Reading Materials

Stress Questionnaires

Perceived Stress Scale (PSS-10), corc.uk.net
https://www.corc.uk.net/outcome-experience-measures/perceived-stress-scale-pss-10/#:~:text=The%20Perceived%20Stress%20Scale%20%28PSS-10%29%20is%20a%2010-item,unpredictable%2C%20uncontrollable%20and%20overloading%20over%20the%20previous%20month.

A Brief Stress Diagnostic Tool: The Short Stress Overload Scale, PubMed (nih.gov)
https://pubmed.ncbi.nlm.nih.gov/30392415/

Boost Your Brain Power! Dr. Heidi Hanna, The Stress Detective
https://heidihanna.com/

Type A and B Personality Model

What is a Type A Personality? The Type A Survival Guide, scienceofpeople.com
https://www.scienceofpeople.com/type-a-personality/

Type A and Type B Personality Theory, Psychology Today United Kingdom
https://www.psychologytoday.com/gb/basics/type-a-and-type-b-personality-theory

What Is a Type A Personality? webmd.com
https://www.webmd.com/balance/what-is-a-type-a-personality

Personality Patterns
Reset Program, alexhoward.com
https://reset.alexhoward.com/

The Five Personality Patterns of Fatigue, What Doctors Don't Tell You (wddty.com)
https://www.wddty.com/features/the-five-personality-patterns-of-fatigue/

The Highly Sensitive Person (HSP) Self Tests, Dr Elain Aaron
https://hsperson.com/test/
The Highly Sensitive Person, Dr Elain Aaron, buy the book, hsperson.com
https://hsperson.com/books/the-highly-sensitive-person/

Neurodivergence and Anxiety

Anxiety Disorders in Adults with Autism Spectrum Disorder: A Population-Based Study, PMC (nih.gov)
https://www.ncbi.nlm.nih.gov/pmc/articles/PMC6946757/

Extending the Minority Stress Model to Understand Mental Health Problems Experienced by the Autistic Population, Monique Botha, David M. Frost, 2020, sagepub.com
https://journals.sagepub.com/doi/10.1177/2156869318804297

New research and free guide: how to adapt mental health talking therapies for autistic children and adults, autism.org.uk
https://www.autism.org.uk/what-we-do/news/adapt-mental-health-talking-therapies

What is neurodiversity? Nicole Baumer, MD, MEd, and Julia Frueh, MD, Harvard Health
https://www.health.harvard.edu/blog/what-is-neurodiversity-202111232645

Neurodiversity and Mental Health, Library News, surrey.ac.uk
https://blogs.surrey.ac.uk/librarynews/2022/03/23/neurodiversity-and-mental-health/

What Does It Mean To Be Neurodivergent? Erin Gregory, Forbes Health
https://www.forbes.com/health/mind/what-is-neurodivergent/

New research and free guide: how to adapt mental health talking therapies for autistic children and adults, autism.org.uk
https://www.autism.org.uk/what-we-do/news/adapt-mental-health-talking-therapies

Book for parents: *Your Child is Not Broken* by Heidi Mavir

ACEs

Adverse childhood experiences: assessing the impact on health and school engagement and the mitigating role of resilience, Christina D Bethell, Paul Newacheck, Eva Hawes, Neal Halfon, PubMed, nih.gov
https://pubmed.ncbi.nlm.nih.gov/25489028/

Adverse childhood experiences and child mental health: an electronic birth cohort study, Emily Lowthian, Rebecca Anthony, Annette Evans, Rhian Daniel, Sara Long, Amrita Bandyopadhyay, Ann John, Mark A. Bellis and Shantini Paranjothy, BMC Medicine, biomedcentral.com
https://bmcmedicine.biomedcentral.com/articles/10.1186/s12916-021-02045-x

Impacts of adverse childhood experiences on health, mental health, and substance use in early adulthood: a cohort study of an urban, minority sample in the U.S, J P Mersky, J Topitzes, A J Reynolds, PubMed, nih.gov
https://pubmed.ncbi.nlm.nih.gov/23978575/

Adverse childhood experiences and mental health in young adults: a longitudinal survey, PubMed, nih.gov
https://pubmed.ncbi.nlm.nih.gov/17343754/

The Impact of Adverse Childhood Experiences on Health and Development in Young Children, Erica M. Webster, 2022, sagepub.com
https://journals.sagepub.com/doi/full/10.1177/2333794X221078708

Part Two
Affirmations

Self-Affirmation Activates Brain Systems Associated with Self-Related Processing and Reward and is Reinforced by Future Orientation, Christopher N. Cascio, Matthew Brook O'Donnell, Francis J Tinney, Matthew Lieberman, researchgate.net
https://www.researchgate.net/publication/283545154_Self-Affirmation_Activates_Brain_Systems_Associated_with_Self-Related_Processing_and_Reward_and_is_Reinforced_by_Future_Orientation

Feeling left out, but affirmed: Protecting against the negative effects of low belonging in college, Kristin Layous, Eden M. Davis, Julio Garcia, Valerie Purdie-Vaughns, Jonathan E. Cook, Geoffrey L. Cohen, kristin-layous.com
http://www.kristinlayous.com/uploads/2/9/2/5/29257173/layous_et_al._2017_-_feeling_left_out_but_affirmed.pdf

Positive Self-Statements: Power for Some, Peril for Others, uni-muenster.de
https://www.uni-muenster.de/imperia/md/content/psyifp/aeechterhoff/wintersemester2011-12/seminarthemenfelderdersozialpsychologie/04_wood_etal_selfstatements_psychscience2009.pdf

Emotions
Diving Deeper Into The Rosenberg Reset, Dr. Joan Rosenberg, drjoanrosenberg.com
https://drjoanrosenberg.com/diving-deeper-into-the-rosenberg-reset/

Book: *Power versus Force* by David R Hawkins

Cold Therapy
How to deal with depression, Wim Hof Method
https://www.wimhofmethod.com/how-to-deal-with-depression

Mindfulness Apps
Best mindfulness apps for kids & teenagers (3), othership.us
https://www.othership.us/resources/best-mindfulness-apps#ch7

Breathwork

Three Breathing Exercises And Techniques, Andrew Weil, M.D., drweil.com
https://www.drweil.com/health-wellness/body-mind-spirit/stress-anxiety/breathing-three-exercises/

Thalamic Gamma Aminobutyric Acid Level Changes in Major Depressive Disorder After a 12-Week Iyengar Yoga and Coherent Breathing Intervention, Chris C. Streeter, MD, Patricia L. Gerbarg, MD, Richard P. Brown, MD, Tammy M. Scott, PhD, Greylin H. Nielsen, BA, Liz Owen, BArch, Osamu Sakai, MD, PhD, Jennifer T. Sneider, PhD, Maren B. Nyer, PhD, and Marisa M. Silveri, PhD, PMC, nih.gov
https://www.ncbi.nlm.nih.gov/pmc/articles/PMC7074898/

3 Steps to Recharge Your Brain and Your Life, Part 1, The Cure for Stress, Heidi Hanna
https://heidihanna.com/2019/04/15/the-cure-for-stress/

Laughter Yoga

Learn Laughter Yoga For Health and Happiness, Laughter Yoga International - Health, Happiness and World Peace
https://www.laughteryoga.org/

Touch

Effects of Gentle Human Touch and Field Massage on Urine Cortisol Level in Premature Infants: A Randomized, Controlled Clinical Trial, Malihe Asadollahi, Mahnaz Jabraeili, Majid Mahallei, Mohammad Asgari Jafarabadi, and Sakine Ebrahimi, PMC, nih.gov
https://www.ncbi.nlm.nih.gov/pmc/articles/PMC5045952/

Physical Contact and Loneliness: Being Touched Reduces Perceptions of Loneliness, A. Heatley Tejada, R. I. M. Dunbar, and M. Montero, PMC, nih.gov
https://www.ncbi.nlm.nih.gov/pmc/articles/PMC7250541/

EFT/Tapping

The Tapping Solution (EFT): How To Get Started
https://www.thetappingsolution.com/

Psychological trauma symptom improvement in veterans using emotional freedom techniques: a randomized controlled trial, Dawson Church, Crystal Hawk, Audrey J Brooks, Olli Toukolehto, Maria Wren, Ingrid Dinter, Phyllis Stein, PubMed, nih.gov
https://pubmed.ncbi.nlm.nih.gov/23364126/

Emotional freedom techniques for treating post traumatic stress disorder: an updated systematic review and meta-analysis, Peta Stapleton, Kevin Kip, Dawson Church, Loren Toussaint, Jacqui Footman, Pat Ballantyne, Tom O'Keefe, frontiersin.org
https://www.frontiersin.org/articles/10.3389/fpsyg.2023.1195286/full?lid=3quhhkbtb7k8

Emotional Freedom Technique (EFT): Tap to relieve stress and burnout, Suzan Blacher, PMC, nih.gov
https://www.ncbi.nlm.nih.gov/pmc/articles/PMC9840127/

Book: *The Tapping Solution* by Nick Ortner

Journalling & Automatic Writing

6 Journaling Benefits and How to Start Right Now, healthline.com
https://www.healthline.com/health/benefits-of-journaling

A Beginners' Guide To Automatic Writing, Kyle Greenfield, The Joy Within
https://thejoywithin.org/empowerment-exercises/automatic-writing

How to Do Automatic Writing, Alexander Peterman, MA, wikiHow
https://www.wikihow.com/Do-Automatic-Writing

Intuitive Painting

What is Intuitive Painting? Creative Juices Arts
https://creativejuicesarts.com/what-is-intuitive-painting/

Food & Diet

Brain Foods for Top Test and Exam Performance, Deane Alban, Be Brain Fit
https://bebrainfit.com/brain-foods-test-exam/

Can food improve your exam performance? **Dr Alex Richardson, BBC Food**
https://www.bbc.co.uk/food/articles/food_exam_performance

Nutritional strategies to ease anxiety, Uma Naidoo, MD, Harvard Health
https://www.health.harvard.edu/blog/nutritional-strategies-to-ease-anxiety-201604139441

Generalized Anxiety Disorder and Hypoglycemia Symptoms Improved with Diet Modification, Monique Aucoin and Sukriti Bhardwaj, PMC, nih.gov
https://www.ncbi.nlm.nih.gov/pmc/articles/PMC4963565/

6 Foods That Trigger Anxiety and What To Eat Instead, Dr Jockers, drjockers.com
https://drjockers.com/6-foods-that-trigger-anxiety-and-what-to-eat-instead/

EXTRA READING MATERIALS

Foods and Drinks Linked to Anxiety: What to Avoid and What to Eat, Ruben Castaneda and Lisa Esposito, U.S. News, usnews.com
https://health.usnews.com/wellness/food/articles/foods-and-drinks-linked-to-anxiety#:~:text=Here%20are%209%20of%20the%20worst%20foods%2C%20drinks,Processed%20meats%2C%20cheese%20and%20ready-made%20meals.%

The 6 Foods You Should Never Eat, Dr. Mark Hyman, drhyman.com
https://drhyman.com/blog/2022/03/14/podcast-ep508/

Foods to Avoid If You Have Anxiety or Depression, Paul Frysh, webmd.com
https://www.webmd.com/depression/ss/slideshow-avoid-foods-anxiety-depression

Anxiety Nutrition Institute
https://www.anxietynutritioninstitute.com/

Book: *Antianxiety Food Solution: of The Antianxiety Food Solution: How the Foods You Eat Can Help You Calm Your Anxious Mind, Improve Your Mood and End Cravings* by Trudy Scott

Sugar

Ultra-Processed Food Consumption and Mental Health: A Systematic Review and Meta-Analysis of Observational Studies, Melissa M. Lane, Elizabeth Gamage, Nikolaj Travica, Thusharika Dissanayaka, Deborah N. Ashtree, Sarah Gauci, Mojtaba Lotfaliany, Adrienne O'Neil, Felice N. Jacka, and Wolfgang Marx, PMC, nih.gov
https://www.ncbi.nlm.nih.gov/pmc/articles/PMC9268228/

The Rats Who Preferred Sugar Over Cocaine, Cynthia Rowland
https://www.cynthiarowland.com/body/the-rats-who-preferred-sugar-over-cocaine/

Sugar intake from sweet food and beverages, common mental disorder and depression: prospective findings from the Whitehall II study, Anika Knüppel, Martin J. Shipley, Clare H. Llewellyn, and Eric J. Brunner, PMC, nih.gov
https://www.ncbi.nlm.nih.gov/pmc/articles/PMC5532289/

Why Your Breakfast Might Be the Perfect Recipe for Stress—and What to Eat Instead, Emily Laurence, wellandgood.com
https://www.wellandgood.com/sugar-and-stress/

The Sugar-Anxiety Connection You Need To Know About, William Cole, IFMCP, DNM, D.C., mindbodygreen
https://www.mindbodygreen.com/articles/why-sugar-might-be-at-the-root-of-your-anxiety?utm_term=pos-1&utm_source=mbg&utm_medium=email&utm_content=&utm_campaign=171004

Caffeine

Caffeine as a Factor Influencing the Functioning of the Human Body—Friend or Foe? Kamil Rodak, Izabela Kokot, and Ewa Maria Kratz, PMC, nih.gov
https://www.ncbi.nlm.nih.gov/pmc/articles/PMC8467199/

Does Drinking Coffee Actually Improve Memory? Elizabeth Hartney, BSc, MSc, MA, PhD, verywellmind.com
https://www.verywellmind.com/does-caffeine-improve-memory-21846

Soda and Fizzy Drinks
Is Soda Bad for Your Brain? (And Is Diet Soda Worse?) Barbara Moran, The Brink, Boston University, bu.edu
https://www.bu.edu/articles/2017/soda-bad-for-brain

Vitamins, Minerals and Herb Supplementation
Controlling Anxiety Through Herbs and Diet, Tess Thompson, anxietyreliefsolutions.com
https://anxietyreliefsolutions.com/controlling-anxiety-through-herbs-and-diet/

Anxiety Natural Remedies: 15 Ways to Relax & Find Calm, Dr Josh Axe, DC, DNM, CN, Dr. Axe, draxe.com
https://draxe.com/health/natural-remedies-anxiety/

B Vitamins

Anxiety Natural Remedies: 15 Ways to Relax & Find Calm, Dr Josh Axe, DC, DNM, CN, Dr. Axe, draxe.com
https://draxe.com/nutrition/vitamin-b6-benefits/

Omega-3 Fatty Acids

Omega-3s for anxiety? Harvard Health
https://www.health.harvard.edu/mind-and-mood/omega-3s-for-anxiety

Can Fish Oil Help Treat Anxiety? Psych Central
https://psychcentral.com/anxiety/fish-oil-for-anxiety

The Importance of Marine Omega-3s for Brain Development and the Prevention and Treatment of Behavior, Mood, and Other Brain Disorders, James J. DiNicolantonio and James H. O'Keefe, PMC, nih.gov
https://www.ncbi.nlm.nih.gov/pmc/articles/PMC7468918/

Magnesium

Association between magnesium intake and depression and anxiety in community-dwelling adults: the Hordaland Health Study, Felice N Jacka, Simon Overland, Robert Stewart, Grethe S Tell, Ingvar Bjelland, Arnstein Mykletun, PubMed, nih.gov
https://pubmed.ncbi.nlm.nih.gov/19085527/

The Effects of Magnesium Supplementation on Subjective Anxiety and Stress—A Systematic Review, Neil Bernard Boyle, Clare Lawton, and Louise Dye, PMC, nih.gov
https://www.ncbi.nlm.nih.gov/pmc/articles/PMC5452159/

Role of magnesium supplementation in the treatment of depression: A randomized clinical trial, Emily K Tarleton, Benjamin Littenberg, Charles D MacLean, Amanda G Kennedy, Christopher Daley, PubMed, nih.gov
https://pubmed.ncbi.nlm.nih.gov/28654669/

Vitamin D

Is Vitamin D Important in Anxiety or Depression? What Is the Truth? Şerife Akpınarcorresponding author and Makbule Gezmen Karadağ, PMC, nih.gov
https://www.ncbi.nlm.nih.gov/pmc/articles/PMC9468237/

Exercise

Regular Physical Activity, Short-Term Exercise, Mental Health, and Well-Being Among University Students: The Results of an Online and a Laboratory Study, Cornelia Herbert, Friedrich Meixner, Christine Wiebking, and Verena Gilg, PMC, nih.gov
https://www.ncbi.nlm.nih.gov/pmc/articles/PMC7264390/

Can exercise help treat anxiety? John J. Ratey, MD, Harvard Health
https://www.health.harvard.edu/blog/can-exercise-help-treat-anxiety-2019102418096

Exercise and Depression, Debra Fulghum Bruce, PhD, webmd.com
https://www.webmd.com/depression/exercise-depression

The anxiolytic effects of exercise: a meta-analysis of randomized trials and dose-response analysis, Bradley M Wipfli, Chad D Rethorst, Daniel M Landers, PubMed, nih.gov
https://pubmed.ncbi.nlm.nih.gov/18723899/

Exercise for anxiety disorders: systematic review, Kaushadh Jayakody, Shalmini Gunadasa, Christian Hosker, PubMed, nih.gov
https://pubmed.ncbi.nlm.nih.gov/23299048/

Exercise and Depression, Debra Fulghum Bruce, PhD, webmd.com
https://www.webmd.com/depression/exercise-depression

Yoga

The effects of yoga on anxiety and stress, Amber W Li, Carroll-Ann W Goldsmith, PubMed, nih.gov
https://pubmed.ncbi.nlm.nih.gov/22502620/

Thalamic Gamma Aminobutyric Acid Level Changes in Major Depressive Disorder After a 12-Week Iyengar Yoga and Coherent Breathing Intervention, Chris C. Streeter, MD, Patricia L. Gerbarg, MD, Richard P. Brown, MD, Tammy M. Scott, PhD, Greylin H. Nielsen, BA, Liz Owen, BArch, Osamu Sakai, MD, PhD, Jennifer T. Sneider, PhD, Maren B. Nyer, PhD, and Marisa M. Silveri, PhD, PMC, nih.gov
https://www.ncbi.nlm.nih.gov/pmc/articles/PMC7074898/

How Yoga Changes Your Brain (It's a Good Thing!), Leah Zerbe, MS, NASM-CPT, NASM-CES, Dr. Axe, draxe.com
https://draxe.com/fitness/how-yoga-changes-your-brain/

Walking In Nature
Effect of phytoncide from trees on human natural killer cell function, Q Li, M Kobayashi, Y Wakayama, H Inagaki, M Katsumata, Y Hirata, K Hirata, T Shimizu, T Kawada, B J Park, T Ohira, T Kagawa, Y Miyazaki, PubMed, nih.gov
https://pubmed.ncbi.nlm.nih.gov/20074458/

Grounding
About Grounding, groundology.co.uk
https://www.groundology.co.uk/about-grounding

The effect of grounding the human body on mood, Gaétan Chevalier, PubMed, nih.gov
https://pubmed.ncbi.nlm.nih.gov/25748085/

Essential Oils
Lavender
A multi-center, double-blind, randomised study of the Lavender oil preparation Silexan in comparison to Lorazepam for generalized anxiety disorder, H Woelk, S Schläfke, PubMed, nih.gov
https://pubmed.ncbi.nlm.nih.gov/19962288/

Lavender and the Nervous System, Peir Hossein Koulivand, Maryam Khaleghi Ghadiri, and Ali Gorji, PMC, nih.gov
https://www.ncbi.nlm.nih.gov/pmc/articles/PMC3612440/

Lemon
The Effectiveness of Aromatherapy for Depressive Symptoms: A Systematic Review, Dalinda Isabel Sánchez-Vidaña, Shirley Pui-Ching Ngai, Wanjia He, Jason Ka-Wing Chow, Benson Wui-Man Lau, and Hector Wing-Hong Tsang, PMC, nih.gov
https://www.ncbi.nlm.nih.gov/pmc/articles/PMC5241490/

Peppermint
Modulation of cognitive performance and mood by aromas of peppermint and ylang-ylang, Mark Moss, Steven Hewitt, Lucy Moss, Keith Wesnes, PubMed, nih.gov
https://pubmed.ncbi.nlm.nih.gov/18041606/

Crystals
The 8 Best Crystal Books For Beginners, Crystal Healing Ritual
https://www.crystalhealingritual.com/crystal-books-for-beginners/

Crystals for Sleep: Catch More Zzz's with These Healing Stones, healthline.com
https://www.healthline.com/health/sleep/crystals-for-sleep

Additional Suicide & Emergency Help
Please find the main contact numbers in the UK under the *Self-Harm and Suicidal Thoughts* section in Part Two of this book.

Signs That Someone Is Contemplating Suicide, Psychology Today United Kingdom
https://www.psychologytoday.com/gb/basics/suicide/warning-signs-of-suicide

Help for suicidal thoughts, NHS, www.nhs.uk
https://www.nhs.uk/mental-health/feelings-symptoms-behaviours/behaviours/help-for-suicidal-thoughts/

Extra Reading Materials

Association for Young People's Health (AYPH), a charity that promotes wellbeing of 10- to 24-year-olds
https://ayph.org.uk/

Charlie Waller Memorial Trust, resources for young people who are depressed
https://www.charliewaller.org/

Family Links, programmes to build resilience, empathy, self esteem, etc. Have specialist programmes working with Islamic values, working with parents in prison or parents of children with disabilities or special needs
https://www.familylinks.org.uk/

Heads Together, mental health campaign to end stigma, supported by the Duke and Duchess of Cambridge and Prince Harry
https://www.headstogether.org.uk/

Hub of Hope, a national database of organisations to access mental health support and advice
https://hubofhope.co.uk/

About the Author

Alison Middleton Timms is an Integrated Wellness Practitioner specialising in mental health, mindset, stress, anxiety and resilience.

A Clinical Hypnotherapist, NLP, EFT, and advanced BLAST Technique® Practitioner and certified health and life coach, Alison is a sought after corporate speaker and trainer, educating and empowering individuals to become the best versions of themselves.

Prior to starting her own business Alison was Former Global Group Head of Talent & Development for Nord Anglia Education and their premium international schools and, before that, spent most of her professional career in top global law firms in various senior HR roles in both London and Hong Kong.

Alison loves being part of the community she lives in. She was a magistrate/JP for years years, is a member of Rotary, Community Champion for her village, and is a volunteer mental health mentor in schools. She lives in Essex and loves spending time out in nature walking, dancing and spending time with family and friends and the family dog, Rosie. She also hosts retreats both in the UK and abroad for those looking to forge deeper connections with themselves. Alison's mantra in life is to make a positive difference on all of those she comes into contact with.

Alison would love to hear how this book has helped you and the tools that have been the most effective for you.

Check out her website at www.amity-health.com

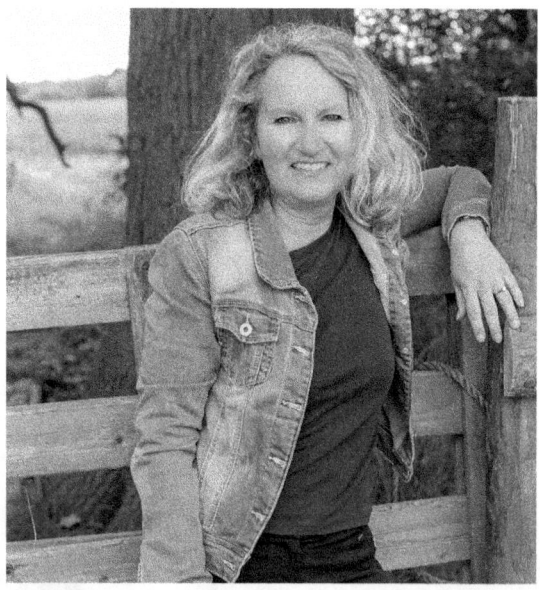

www.ingramcontent.com/pod-product-compliance
Lightning Source LLC
Chambersburg PA
CBHW051541020426
42333CB00016B/2034